SHARKS
DON'T GET
CANCER

SHARKS
DON'T GET
CANCER

DR. I. WILLIAM LANE
LINDA COMAC

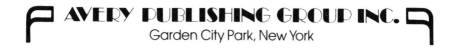
AVERY PUBLISHING GROUP INC.
Garden City Park, New York

The advice in this book is based on the training of, experiences of, and pool of information available to the authors. Mention of any research organization or individual researcher should in no way be construed as an endorsement of this book or of any techniques therein. Because each person and situation are unique, the editor and the publisher urge the reader to check with a qualified health professional when there is any question regarding the presence or treatment of any abnormal health condition. The publisher does not advocate the use of any particular treatment but believes the information in this book should be available to the public.

Because there is always some risk involved, the author and publisher are not responsible for any adverse effects or consequences resulting from the use of any of the preparations or procedures described in this book. Please do not use this book if you are unwilling to assume the risk. For personalized advice, please consult a physician or other qualified health professional. It is a sign of wisdom, not cowardice, to seek a second or third opinion.

Cover Design: Rudy Shur and Janine Eisner-Wall
In-House Editors: Elaine Will Sparber and Joanne Abrams
Typesetter: Bonnie Freid

Publisher's Cataloging in Publication

Lane, I. William.
 Sharks don't get cancer : how shark cartilage could save your life / I. William Lane, Linda Comac.
 p. cm.
 Includes bibliographical references and index.
 ISBN 0-89529-520-2

 1. Cancer—Prevention. 2. Neovascularization. 3. Sharks. I. Comac, Linda. II. Title.

RC271.S53L3 1992   616.994'052
 QBI92-782

Printed in the United States of America

20 19

Contents

This book is dedicated:

To all those who are willing to look beyond that which is considered the norm; to those people—both professional and lay—who have risked ridicule, loss of status, condemnation by peers, and sometimes even legal persecution in order to go that extra mile and possibly alter the status quo.

To those scientists who develop new theories, such as the theory that is the basis of this book, a theory developed by the eminent New England scientist Dr. Judah Folkman, as well as Dr. Robert Langer and Dr. Patricia D'Amore, for whom I have the utmost respect.

To open-minded research scientists the world over, especially the four mentioned in this book who, in the European city of Brussels, were willing to run with an idea brought to them in its infancy. Their attitudes and cooperation have allowed that idea to advance and mature on solid ground.

To a distinguished cancer research scientist—an American of Belgian heritage who prefers to remain unnamed—who recognized the potential of and guided the early work with shark cartilage.

Finally, to the memory of Sis, Helen, and Maggie—and the countless other victims of cancer—for whom this information on shark cartilage came too late.

Permissions

The quotes from Dr. Patricia D'Amore on pages 1, 41, and 49–50 have been reprinted with permission from *Seminars in Thrombosis and Hemostasis* 14:73–77 © 1988 by Thieme Medical Publishers, Inc.

The quotes from Dr. Judah Folkman on pages 1, 56, and 61 have been reprinted with permission from "Antiangiogenesis" in *Biologic Therapy of Cancer*, edited by Vincent T. DeVita, Jr., M.D., Samuel Hellman, M.D., and Steven A. Rosenberg, M.D., © 1991 by J. B. Lippincott Company.

The quote from Warren E. Leary on page 37 has been reprinted with the permission of the Associated Press.

The quote from Dr. John Prudden on page 48 has been reprinted with permission from "The Treatment of Human Cancer With Agents Prepared From Bovine Cartilage," *Journal of Biological Response Modifiers* 4:551–584, 1985.

The quotes from Dr. Noel Weidner *et al.* on pages 53 and 55 have been excerpted with permission from information appearing in *The New England Journal of Medicine* 324:1–8, 1991.

The quotes from Arnold I. Caplan on pages 113 and 144 have been reprinted with permission from *Scientific American* 251:84–94, © 1984 by Scientific American, Inc. All rights reserved.

The quotes from Dr. John Prudden on pages 115 and 129 have been reprinted with permission from *Seminars in Arthritis and Rheumatism* 3:287–321, 1974.

The quote from V. Rejholee on page 118 has been reprinted with permission from *Seminars in Arthritis and Rheumatism* 17:35–63, 1987.

The quotes from Thomas H. Maugh III on pages 134–135 have been reprinted with permission from *Science* 212:1374–1375, © 1981 by the American Association for the Advancement of Science.

The quote from Dr. Louis Lasagna on page 147 has been reprinted with permission from the "Final Report of the National Committee to Review Current Procedures for Approval of New Drugs for Cancer and AIDS."

Acknowledgments

Sincere thanks go to all the people at Avery Publishing Group. Without them, this book would never have become a reality.

Special thanks to Rudy Shur, managing editor, whose belief in the need for this book and in the "power of the people" was a driving force behind this work.

And a very warm thank you to Elaine Will Sparber and Joanne Abrams, editors, for their patience, grace under pressure, and commitment to excellence.

Thanks, too, to Roger Jacobs, Ph.D., for his support, technical advice, computer acumen, and belief that a scientist's job is to find the truth.

Foreword

How many funerals have you attended this year for friends or family members who died of cancer?

If you observed these loved ones undergoing the torture of conventional cancer treatments, you can understand how overjoyed I was years ago when I discovered the world of alternative cancer therapies. These nontoxic therapies designed to strengthen the patient's immune system have, in many cases, cured cancer patients or extended their lives and improved their quality of life.

But what discourages and frustrates me as a health writer investigating nontoxic cancer treatments is the refusal on the part of the cancer establishment to investigate promising cancer treatments that originate outside the establishment. Instead, the National Cancer Institute (NCI) and other government agencies prefer to label such treatments "unproven," a euphemism for "quackery."

In their efforts to discredit a promising treatment, members of the medical establishment have no compunction about ignoring scientific evidence, as my husband discovered when his articles about the Heimlich maneuver appeared in leading medical journals in the mid-1970s. Reports came from all over the country about choking persons being saved by the maneuver, but the American Red Cross derided the reports as "anecdotal" and continued for ten years to teach backslapping, which causes the stuck object to lodge even tighter in the throat of the choking victim.

This hostility on the part of the establishment towards alternative cancer treatments stems, in part, from the NIH ("not invented here") mindset. How can the NCI justify its yearly budget of $1.4 billion if a cure for cancer originates elsewhere? In addition, another strike against alternative cancer treatments is these treatments' use of natural substances. A natural substance (whether a whole food, natural enema, or vitamin supplement) cannot be patented, leaving the pharmaceutical companies, which support vast amounts of medical research, with no interest in funding studies on the substance. Government research organizations and university hospitals are all closely allied with the pharmaceutical industry.

Enter shark cartilage, a natural nontoxic substance that has been shown to inhibit tumor growth, as evidenced by published laboratory studies conducted by eminent scientists over a thirty-year period. And, if the studies proving that shark cartilage is an effective cancer treatment and preventive were not sufficient cause for rejoicing, these studies also indicate that a substance in shark cartilage has the potential to control arthritis, psoriasis, macular degeneration, and other diseases of aging.

Sounds like the breakthrough of the century, doesn't it? Except, knowing what you now know about the old boys' club in medicine and the power of the pharmaceutical industry, I think you'll agree that the odds of shark cartilage being tested, let alone accepted, by the medical establishment are slim indeed.

So, shark cartilage might easily have remained buried in the scientific journals if I. William Lane, Ph.D., had not stumbled on the scene. Lane, a colorful mix of marine expert, nutritionist, and international businessman, could hardly believe what he found in the ivory towers. How Lane almost single-handedly made shark cartilage available to you as a food supplement is part of this enthralling medical detective story. You'll learn the scientific rationale that explains why shark cartilage has such potential as a treatment for so many "incurable" diseases. You'll also get a rare glimpse into our health-care system, the "most profitable industry" in the United States.

But most important, if you have cancer or wish to prevent a recurrence, or if you suffer from arthritis or another disabling disease, or if you are healthy and wish to remain so, *Sharks Don't Get Cancer* may provide the information you need to significantly improve your health.

Jane Heimlich
Author of *What Your Doctor Won't Tell You*

Preface

Have you ever noticed something that no one else did? Even though it's right there, in front of everyone's nose, few people seem to pay much attention to it. For you, on the other hand, it stands out like a great big red neon sign. And once you've noticed it, nothing else looks quite the same. What you've seen has changed the direction of your life.

Back in 1983, I saw something that I believed could change the course of cancer therapy. I was fortunate enough to have a unique combination of scientific background and business experience that enabled me to see opportunities apparently no one else saw.

My education in nutrition, biochemistry, and agriculture led to my involvement with the fishing industry, which I eventually served in research, management, and operations capacities. In the late 1970s, I became particularly interested in the development of shark fishing as an industry. Along the way, and quite by accident, I found out about a theory published by some very learned and respected scientists but not made known to the general public. *Sharks Don't Get Cancer* was written in the belief that information about the therapeutic and prophylactic potential of products derived from sharks, information that has already generated a great deal of excitement among researchers, should be available to the public at large.

It has become my single-minded purpose to get others—professionals and laypeople alike—involved in studies that I feel will lead to the control and prevention of some of the most devastating illnesses known to man. To achieve my ends, I've chosen to travel a road that others, perhaps, have traveled but have been forced to abandon, and although I've given up a great deal to pursue this path, I would do it again. Hopefully, my work will help health-care professionals understand that natural products have the potential to do a heck of a lot of good. I hope they will see that these products have been largely ignored while investigators look for the so-called magic bullet.

I've brought my work to you in *Sharks Don't Get Cancer*, although I must admit that *some* sharks do get cancer. The number is, however, insignificant; and while *ALMOST No Sharks Get Cancer* might have been a bit more accurate, it would have been a rotten title.

I'll begin my book by introducing you to the "hero" of the story—perhaps of the century. You'll learn all about the shark—a most successful animal—in Chapter 1. Then, in Chapter 2, we'll look at the over twenty years of research leading up to this book, beginning with a Harvard researcher's theory of angiogenesis. An overview of what the traditional researchers have been doing is followed, in Chapter 3, by the story of my own involvement in the research, with particular emphasis on bringing the research to the clinical-trial stage. In describing my activities and the various activities of others, *Sharks Don't Get Cancer* asks why it has taken over two decades for potentially lifesaving information to reach the general public.

In Chapter 4, you'll find out that among researchers, clinicians, and informed members of the public, excitement continues to mount about shark cartilage. Clinical trials on women with breast, cervical, uterine, and other deadly cancers are underway; new cancer research projects with animals and humans are being undertaken on an almost daily basis in the United States, France, Germany, and Holland. Clinical work using cartilage to alleviate the pain associated with arthritis in dogs and in humans has already been published in the scientific literature. Studies done to date have been motivated purely by excitement over the possibilities; researchers have received no recompense for their efforts.

In Chapter 5, you'll discover that *Sharks Don't Get Cancer* is a title that reflects only the tip of the iceberg. Sharks may also prove instrumental in the prevention and cure of some of man's other dreaded diseases, diseases against which modern medicine has been largely ineffective, diseases in which the procedures used are often quite devastating, with results and side effects that are sometimes more destructive than the diseases themselves.

Every attempt has been made to make this book easy for a nonscientific audience to understand. Those readers wishing more detailed and scientific explanations of the research being done will find an extensive bibliography at the end of the volume. The bibliography also documents the extent and caliber of the research into angiogenesis and its effects on cancer and other degenerative diseases. For the compilation of a large part of this bibliography, I am indebted to Norman Ackerman, M.D., Ph.D., professor of surgery at New York Medical College in Westchester County and recently retired chief of surgery at Metropolitan Hospital Center in New York City. Dr. Ackerman graciously made available the files he had amassed while planning his own research into the inhibition of angiogenesis.

A glossary has been provided for those readers who are in doubt about any of the terms used in the book. Readers will also find boxed insets scattered throughout the text. These insets provide more information about some of the subjects mentioned in the book.

When you have finished reading *Sharks Don't Get Cancer*, you will understand why malignant tumors are rarely, if ever, found in sharks and how this fact may potentially be used to save your life or the life of someone you love. Both open-minded professionals and laypersons will quickly comprehend how shark cartilage can be used in the cure and treatment, and probably the prevention, of many dreaded diseases. The approach holds little to no risk for most adults, is simple to understand, and can be used along with other approaches that health professionals may wish to follow.

If you are one of the scores of people who have come to believe that cancer research in the United States seems to be getting nowhere; if you are one of those who have watched someone suffer through chemotherapy or radiation and die anyway; if you are a medical practitioner or researcher who believes that there must be a better way, then *Sharks Don't Get Cancer* has information you'll want.

Dr. I. William Lane
Millburn, New Jersey

. . . antiangiogenic therapy could restrict the growth of a wide variety of solid tumors while being administered for prolonged periods, with low toxicity and a low probability of drug resistance.

M. Judah Folkman, M.D.
Harvard Medical School
Biologic Therapy of Cancer

The only event that stands between maintenance of metastatic cells in a dormant state and their establishment into a secondary tumor is the development of a vasculature [system of blood vessels]. Thus therapies aimed at interfering with vascularization represent viable strategies for antimetastasis.

Patricia A. D'Amore, Ph.D.
Harvard Medical School
Seminars in Thrombosis and Hemostasis

Introduction

More than 1 million people in the United States were diagnosed with cancer in 1990. Cancer, which is now the second leading cause of death in the United States, claims more than 500,000 lives each year. Basing its estimates on statistics, the American Cancer Society projects that approximately 76 million Americans now living will eventually develop cancer. It also predicts that by the year 2000, about 1 out of every 2 people will develop the disease—that's 1 out of every 2 in just a few years' time!

In sharp contrast, the cancer rate for sharks is estimated to be 1 out of 1 million or even less. That's quite a difference, a difference that has led a handful of scientists to believe that within the shark itself lies the secret to curing and preventing most major forms of cancer.

A prehistoric creature that has existed largely unchanged for more than 400 million years, the shark is one of the few beings on Earth that rarely if ever get cancer. Only seven tumors were reported to have been found in sharks prior to the establishment of the Registry of Tumors in Lower Animals by the Smithsonian Institution in 1965. More recently, staff members at the registry conducted a computer search of existing records and discovered that in 4,500 published reports on sharks and approximately 3,000 museum specimens, there were only thirty shark tumors mentioned; more than half of these were considered to be "incorrect diagnoses." Researchers who study elasmobranchs (sharks, skates, and rays) have rarely—if ever—reported finding malignancies during the autopsies they performed on thousands of sharks. The total number of shark tumors is less than a fraction of 1 percent of the total tumors reported for all fishes.

Scientists who wanted to find out why sharks so rarely develop cancer asked, "What is so different about a shark that might cause this phenomenon?" The answer to this question is part of a discovery that may prove to be the most momentous medical breakthrough of the century, a discovery that touches upon cancer and a host of degenerative diseases that haunt modern man such as arthritis, an inflammation of the joints; enteritis, an inflammation of the intestinal tract; diabetic retinopathy, an eye disorder in which small blood vessels of the retina dilate and rupture; and psoriasis, a disease of the skin. These diseases have more in common than may appear at first glance. They are all conditions against which modern medicine has not done well, and some are diseases associated with aging—a major problem for a society in which the average age has steadily been rising. Now, new evidence reveals that they are also all angiogenesis-based conditions—conditions dependent upon the growth of new blood vessels.

IN PURSUIT OF A CURE

Sharks Don't Get Cancer begins—as did most of the shark-cartilage research being conducted today—with a theory developed by world-renowned scientist and Harvard professor Dr. Judah Folkman. More than twenty years ago, Dr. Folkman showed that tumor growth could be restricted to the size of a pencil point. Subsequent work at the Massachusetts Institute of Technology (MIT) by Dr. Robert Langer and Dr. Anne Lee laid the second cornerstone of the development, the cornerstone that brought sharks into the scenario for a possible cancer cure. Scientists, you see, have long known that sharks do not develop cancer, whether they are bred in clean open waters or in carcinogen-laden enclosed waters. For years, a scientist in Sarasota, Florida, has been putting sharks into tanks containing strong concentrations of carcinogens (cancer-causing agents); for years, he has been unable to produce a single tumor in a shark.

According to the most recent statistics, the amount now spent on health care in the United States has reached 12 percent of the Gross National Product (GNP)—over $700 *billion*—at least twice that spent by any other country and three times that spent by Japan. It is estimated that the expenditure will climb to 14 percent of the GNP by 1993. Of this immense outlay, only 3 percent is used for preventative applications, while 92 percent is used for treatment after the patient is already ill. Preventative therapy and practice, proper diet, and a clean environment may be the only logical means to control spiraling health costs—costs that are measured in billions of dollars, quality of life, and life itself.

Imagine, then, the far-reaching effects of a natural nontoxic product that acts both as a therapeutic agent and as a prophylactic (protective measure). That's what *Sharks Don't Get Cancer* is all about. It is the story of a simple observation, a brilliant theory, and a practical application of that theory, which, when combined, may save the lives of untold millions as well as relieve the pain and suffering of millions more.

1.

The Shark

The sea's living resources will and should be harvested and sharks, out of necessity, will doubtless be among them.

Thomas H. Lineaweaver III
and Richard H. Backus
The Natural History of Sharks

Dinosaurs once stalked the land. Pterodactyl winged their way across the sky. However, more than 200 million years before these creatures held dominion over land and sky, sharks swam in the seas. And though the dinosaurs have vanished, the shark—probably the longest-lived animal on Earth—is still with us.

Sharks are among the most primitive of any living vertebrates, untouched by the forces of evolution. They have survived, and remained largely unchanged, for 400 million years simply because they are the creatures best suited for survival—perfectly outfitted in their structure, their senses, their mating habits, and their resistance to disease. In addition, sharks' only predators are other sharks and human beings, although porpoises are sometimes considered sharks' enemies. (See "Sharks and Porpoises" on page 9.)

Many of the adaptations that have enabled the shark to long endure also enable individual shark species to be long-lived, attaining life spans that range from twenty-five to one hundred years. It is believed that the spiny dogfish, for instance, lives seventy years, perhaps even a whole century. There is more concrete information about the well-known Australian school shark, which has been fished for more than half a century. Tagging of these sharks revealed several that were about sixty years old.

What are the unique characteristics of the shark that have enabled it to survive when other animals have vanished? Are there things we can learn from the shark—or perhaps even *take* from the shark—that will give people some of the same characteristics, enabling us to live longer or healthier lives?

In seeking the answers to these questions, we need to begin by considering what is known about sharks.

NOT A BONE IN THEIR BODIES

The most obvious difference between sharks and any other land or water creature is the absence of bone. That's right; a shark doesn't have a single bone in its body. Most animals, including man, have skeletons composed of calcified bone. The skeletons of sharks are made of pure cartilage, a hard gristly material formed from proteins and complex carbohydrates and toughened by rodlike fibers. (See "What Is This Thing Called Cartilage?" on page 11.)

Sharks belong to the ancient class of *Elasmobranchii*, which derives its name from the same Greek root as does the word *elastic—el*, meaning "to cause to go." Indeed, the nonrigid body of the shark appears almost elastic in motion. Less dense and more pliable than bone, cartilage provides the shark with the advantages of buoyancy and flexibility. There is, however, at

Sharks and Porpoises

"Although almost anything may be found inside sharks, sharks are not often found inside anything except other sharks," write Thomas H. Lineaweaver III and Richard H. Backus in their book "The Natural History of Sharks." Sharks, being cannibals, will eat others of their kind, but the only other creature known to eat sharks is the human animal. Even whales, which have the jaw and tooth power to eat a shark, do not do so. It appears then that sharks have no natural enemies except man and other sharks. But what about the porpoise, which has been known to kill sharks by butting them to death?

For the most part, sharks and porpoises leave each other alone and are even, on occasion, seen feeding together. Sharks will, however, eat porpoises and are often found with the remains of the gentle animal in their stomachs. Porpoises cannot, on the other hand, eat sharks. Their jaws and teeth are simply not strong enough. Porpoises are then enemies of sharks, but they are not predators of sharks.

The relationship between the species is graphically illustrated by Lineaweaver and Backus' account of a fishing boat's encounter with the two sea creatures. A slow-moving fishing boat was once surrounded by about fifty porpoises that appeared to be exhausted and injured. Older porpoises were patrolling the outer ring of the circle of animals, while six or so young porpoises were being herded close to the boat. The fishermen on board the boat soon noted that there were several sharks swimming about thirty yards away from the porpoises. The "patrol" porpoises would burst into a series of dashes if a shark came near. Apparently, the boat was being used to protect one flank of the group of porpoises.

The fishermen were troubled that they could do nothing to help the porpoises. Stopping the boat only seemed to draw the sharks in closer. Eventually, a brief, violent rainstorm obscured the activity in the water, and when the storm ended, the fishermen discovered that all the animals had gone.

For many years, the fishermen talked of the cooperation among the porpoises and of the porpoises' concentrated effort to protect their young.

least one disadvantage to the lack of bone. Because a shark does not have a rigid skeleton or a rib cage to protect its internal organs, it can be killed by a porpoise—one of its normal food sources—in a one-on-one fight. The porpoise can literally butt the shark to death since there is no rigid rib cage to protect the shark's vital organs.

Bone's rigidity and ability to protect vital organs are not the only ways in which it differs from cartilage. Bone is composed primarily of calcium and phosphorus salts. Cartilage does not usually contain these salts, nor does it contain the microscopic canals that in bone permit the passage of blood vessels and nerve fibers. Cartilage has no blood vessels or nerves, whereas bone does.

Bone and cartilage do have some similarities, however. Both begin to form in the middle layer of the embryo, where the cells will subsequently develop as either cartilage, bone, or connective tissue. In addition, both bone and cartilage contain collagen, the main supportive protein of skin and tendon as well as cartilage and bone.

Between 6 and 8 percent of a shark's gross weight is cartilage; only a small fraction of 1 percent of a mammal's gross weight is cartilage. In humans, for instance, cartilage is found in the harder parts of the ears and nose, around joints, at the ends of long bones, and between the segments of the spine. In

What Is This Thing Called Cartilage?

We break our bones, tear our ligaments, strain our muscles. What do we do to our cartilage? What—where, in fact—is cartilage?

You're probably most familiar with cartilage as the "tough stuff" that you don't want in your meat, but when eating, you most likely refer to it as "gristle." Cartilage is apparent in the human body, too, but we call it by other names, such as "Adam's apple," a translation from the Hebrew "tappuah haadam."

Cartilage is found not only in the larynx but also between the segments of the spine and at the ends of long bones, where it acts as a shock absorber and a bearing surface to reduce the friction between moving parts. It is a tough, elastic, and translucent material that comes in three varieties.

Fibrocartilage, the first variety, is found between the backbones. It is the strongest of the three types. The second, hyaline cartilage, is gristly elastic tissue that thinly covers the moving ends of bones, connects the ribs to the breastbone, and supports the nose, windpipe, and part of the voice box. This type of cartilage is likely to harden in elderly people. Yellow cartilage, the third variety, is the most elastic. It is found in the external ear, Eustachian tube, and throat.

One of the most interesting things about cartilage, however, is not its form but its importance to the body, an importance that is first apparent in the embryo.

Embryonic Development

In an early fetus, there are no bones; it is cartilage that provides the framework on which the major bones of the body—excluding the skull—take form. Eventually, fetal cartilage becomes impregnated with calcium salts so that hard, or "stony," bones become apparent.

The bones of children are relatively pliable because they contain more cartilage—which is found at the tops of bones in zones called growth plates—and less calcium salts than do the bones of adults. (A theory has been postulated that newborn children are resistant to many diseases because of the large amount of cartilage present in their bodies during the early fetal and developmental stages.) Elderly people have much less soft tissue such as cartilage and a higher proportion of calcium salts, so their bones are more brittle.

A process similar to the one in which fetal cartilage develops into bone takes place throughout life whenever bones are broken. It is believed that when a bone breaks, a substance within the bone signals cells from the circulatory system to clean out the breakage site and summon undifferentiated cells to populate the site and multiply. These undifferentiated cells become chondrocytes, or cartilage cells, which produce an intertwining of cartilaginous fibers that fills the break and joins the bone fragments together. Finally, the cartilage is calcified and becomes new living bone.

Amazingly, cartilage is a tissue that performs its functions without nerves, blood vessels, or a lymphatic system. Nutrients are, therefore, not transported to cartilage via the blood or lymphatic fluid. It is the flow of water, the chief constituent of cartilage, that is responsible for nutrient transport, which is brought on by the compressions and relaxations arising from body movements. This is why extended periods of inactivity are deleterious to joint cartilage.

As a result of inactivity, the calcium salts in cartilage's intercellular material can turn from a water-containing gel into a stonelike material. The calcification cannot be reversed or repaired as can torn ligaments or broken bones. Calcification is ultimately the death of cartilage.

an average calf—a mammal whose weight is roughly equivalent to that of an average shark—cartilage is only 0.06 percent of the total body weight. This means a shark has 1,000 times as much cartilage as does a calf or other similar-sized mammal.

In addition to sharks having a higher percentage of cartilage than mammals, sharks' cartilage is also different in that it has some calcification. Shark cartilage is reinforced at stress points with plates of apatite, a substance composed of calcium phosphates and carbonates. In the cartilage of most animals, such calcification is usually limited to the surface areas of cartilage, but shark vertebrae must withstand the stresses associated with the motions of swimming and therefore are often reinforced.

Lack of a calcified skeleton means that the shark does not have a backbone the way most fishes do. However, the shark does have a spinal column, which is made of cartilage and extends into and supports the upper part of the tail. The shark's skeleton is divided into two parts—the axial portion, which includes the skull and vertebral column, and the appendicular portion, which includes the pectoral and pelvic girdles and median fin cartilages, which provide support for the fins (see Figure 1.1). The cartilaginous fins enhance the shark's swimming ability.

Sharks usually swim at three to five miles per hour and cannot stop quickly or back up. Their boneless bodies must bend and curve to turn back, actions that are facilitated by the strong tails and fins. Sharks have two sets of paired fins, but it is the large, triangular dorsal fin on the top of the shark's body and the flag-shaped tail that are so distinct. All the fins are relatively inflexible and are used for steering, stabilization, and propulsion. The pectoral fins, with their wide spread, and the tail fin, with its upward curve, provide the lift; the tail, with its sweeping movement, provides the drive. This arrangement is what gives sharks their excellent swimming ability, which is so vital to their survival.

Sharks must be constantly on the move in order to live and to keep from sinking; some varieties never even sleep. Like all living creatures, sharks need oxygen; like all fishes, sharks get

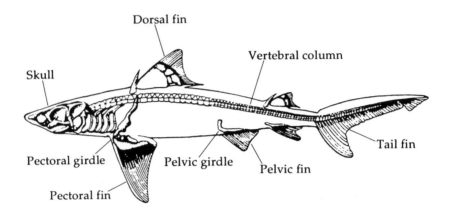

Figure 1.1. An artist's rendering of a shark shows the parts of the cartilaginous skeleton.

their oxygen from air contained in the water. Many sharks must keep swimming in order to force the water through their gills. They can stop swimming only in a rapidly moving water current that will push the water into their gills. Bony fishes use their mouths and gill covers as pumps, opening and closing them to force the water through the gills.

In addition to the vertebrae and fins of the shark being composed of cartilage, the shark's skull is also made of cartilage, although, here again, deposits of mineral salts make the skull very hard. In the skull are housed the brain and sense organs. Perhaps more than anything else, the sense organs, which are incredibly developed, set the shark apart as a successful—and terrifying—creature.

SENSES

The shark's unique sense organs are invaluable aids to food-gathering. Each of the shark's senses comes into play at a different point in the hunt, ensuring that the prey cannot sneak by. The shark's hearing can be measured in thousands of yards; the shark's sense of smell (olfaction), in hundreds of yards. The vision of a shark is limited to about fifty feet, and touch and taste obviously require contact. All the sense organs work together to make the shark a feared hunter.

Ampullae of Lorenzini

Perhaps the most amazing of the sense organs are the ampullae of Lorenzini, which the shark utilizes just inches from its victim. These small bundles of sensory cells are located under the skin around the head. They are composed almost entirely of nerve fibers and detect weak electrical fields at short ranges, enabling sharks to find prey even without visual or olfactory clues. In addition, a series of fluid-filled canals lies just beneath the skin of the head and along the sides of the body. This "lateral line" and the ampullae of Lorenzini along with an internal ear constitute a complex system of receptors that transforms underwater sound or mechanical disturbance into nerve impulses, allowing sharks to home in on a particular motion or sound.

Hearing

The shark's highly sensitive hearing may be its first means of detecting prey. Sound travels faster and farther in water than it does in air, and sharks are drawn to irregular, low-frequency vibrations at distances of more than a mile. Pure and continuous sounds do not seem to attract a shark's attention, probably because such sounds are more likely to be made by a freely swimming animal than by a wounded one. Sharks hear sounds ranging from 100 cycles per second (about one octave below the high end of a piano) to about 1,500 cycles per second (about two octaves above the low end of a piano). These sounds become less important to the hunt as the shark gets closer to its prey.

Olfaction

Once a shark is within several hundred yards of its prey, its olfactory ability comes into play. Smell, one of the most important of the shark's senses, is celebrated in folklore and cinema for good reason. The average eight-foot shark has a brain that is seven inches long. Two-thirds of the brain's weight is dedicated to the olfactory function. In addition, the nostrils of a shark do not communicate with the mouth and have no function in breathing; they are solely olfactory. Sharks can smell blood a mile away, especially in a current. They can sense one drop of blood in a million gallons of water; they can, in other words, smell a half teaspoon of blood in three swimming pools' worth of water. This, combined with their ability to hear the abnormal beat of an old or hurt fish half a mile away, makes sharks the perfect scavengers, feeding primarily on wounded fish.

In one experiment to test the shark's olfactory abilities, a shark was put into a tank with a crab. The shark swam in ever smaller circles till it grabbed the crab. When crabs were wrapped in cheesecloth and placed in the tank along with stones wrapped in cheesecloth, the shark grabbed the crabs and ignored the stones. However, when the shark's nasal capsules were plugged, the shark ignored the crabs even when they were directly offered to it.

The typical zigzag swimming pattern of a shark on the hunt is also testimony to its acute sense of smell. The shark picks up a scent and begins to swim toward it. If the shark is heading to the left of its prey, the right nostril picks up the scent, so the shark swings to the right. Now its left nostril picks up the scent, causing it to veer again. When a shark is not tracking a scent, it swims in a more direct path. The zigzag swimming movement—a mirror of the saw-edged teeth of the shark—is, like the teeth, something of which to be wary.

Vision

As the shark begins its final approach toward its prey, vision takes over from the sense of smell. The sense of sight is the most important hunting tool from the time the shark is about fifty feet from its prey up to the actual moment of attack. This was demonstrated in an experiment in which four-inch cubes of fish and four-inch cubes of wood were dropped three feet from a shark. In twenty trials over a two-day period, the shark grabbed the fish eleven times and the wood nine times. Apparently, the shark could not "sniff out" any difference at such a short distance.

The eye of the shark is uniquely outfitted for a life of hunting. Sensitive eyes are set far apart, one on each side of the head, an especially recognizable attribute of the hammerhead shark. The eye muscles allow the eyeball to rotate so that the field of vision is constant whether the shark is turning or swimming in a straight line. The eyes detect differences in light and darkness because they contain many rods, the cells that are sensitive to dim light. In some sharks, a specialized group of cells helps to protect the rods from possible damage by bright light. In bright light, these cells, which have a black pigment, move into place almost like blinds. In dim light, the cells retire.

In addition, a shark's eye has a mirror-like layer, called the tapetum lucidum, behind the retina. Crystals in this layer reflect light that has already passed through the retina, stimulating the retina a second time and making it more efficient under low-light conditions. Some sharks also have a nictitating membrane that protects the eye from mechanical injury.

The nictitating membrane is a second lower eyelid that is

extended over the eye at the moment of biting or when the shark passes close to objects. This fills in the gap between the upper and lower eyelids, which are mobile but do not completely cover the eyeball. Recent developments in close-up camera work have allowed us to see that the shark is actually blind at the moment of attack. For protection from the sharp teeth and nails of struggling prey, the eyeball rotates back in its socket. The shark must therefore rely on the ampullae of Lorenzini during close-range hunting. At the moment when the shark bites, the ampullae may be the controlling sensory apparatus.

The sense organs of the shark work in unison so that the shark can easily track its prey. During the last moments, the senses of touch and taste help the shark determine whether it will devour its meal or not. At this time, the powerful teeth and jaws go to work.

TEETH AND JAWS

The jaws and teeth of the shark are rightfully famous—or infamous. The mouth, situated behind a long snout, is crescent-shaped, curving backward to create the savage snarl of cartoon fame. In cartoon, cinema, and reality, the shark's teeth and jaws often leave bloody evidence of their frequently fatal danger.

A shark's teeth are well adapted to its diet, varying in shape according to the specific species' main food. It is, in fact, the shape of the teeth that classifies the shark—white sharks have triangular teeth with jagged edges; blue pointers have large pointed fangs; sand and tiger sharks have ragged teeth. The variations in size, shape, number, and arrangement of sharks' teeth make it possible for an ichthyologist (one who studies fishes) to identify a species from a single tooth.

Generally speaking, a shark's teeth are arranged along the borders of the upper and lower jaws. They are used for seizing, cutting, piercing, and crunching. Situated along the gums are four complete sets of fully developed replacement teeth, which move forward as the front row of teeth wears out. As the front row of teeth crumbles and the second row moves forward to take its place, a new fifth row of teeth grows in at the back. In 1966, it was discovered that the teeth in the upper jaw of a young shark are replaced every 7.2 days; the teeth in the lower jaw, every 8.2 days. A shark can use up more than 20,000 teeth in ten years because the considerable biting force exerted by the jaws often damages the teeth.

The shark's jaws are hinged, with the upper jaw rather loosely fitted so that its reach can be extended. These are the most powerful jaws in the world. A metal scale wrapped inside bait revealed that an eight-foot shark has a bite pressure of 18 tons per square inch. When a Snodgrass Gnathodynamometer was used to measure the force exerted by the jaws, it registered 6,613.8 pounds per square centimeter.

FACT OR FICTION?

A shark's jaws obviously have tremendous power. But many other aspects of "sharklore" are more fiction than fact. People have, for instance, become accustomed to thinking about the shark as a dangerous man-eater cruising the ocean's surface with his dorsal fin showing. This triangle of terror spreads fear among sailors and landlubbers alike. In actual fact, the largest shark populations are found near the bottom, not the surface, of the ocean, so a fin that breaks the surface is more likely to belong to a ray than to a shark.

Despite what you may have heard, the shark is not man's natural enemy. Sharks evolved millions of years before man; therefore, the shark's diet never included human flesh. Man can be considered only, as José Castro, author of *The Sharks of North American Waters*, puts it, "accidental prey."

Although sharks do not seek out human beings and usually will flee from people, they are scavengers and are curious and often hungry. This may account for their gruesome reputation, a reputation whose beginnings can possibly be traced to the Bible. Many scholars have claimed that Jonah was swallowed by a shark—a great white shark—rather than a whale. One of the earliest of these references is found in Heinrich Herman Frey's 1594 *Biblisch Fischbuch* (*Biblical Fish Book*).

Another common misconception about sharks is that they scavenge for rotten flesh. This is not the case. Indeed, the whale shark—the largest of all fishes—consumes only small living animals and plants, straining them from the water through its teeth. Both whale sharks and basking sharks swim lazily at speeds of two to three miles per hour with their mouths wide open. Tons of water carrying food flow through their jaws. Their gill rakers act as strainers, keeping the food in and allowing the strained water to pass on through the gills. A 23-foot basking shark can strain 4 million pounds of sea water in one hour.

Although these large shark species do not attack people, there are a small number of species that do engage in unprovoked attacks on humans. It is the white shark—the third largest fish in the world—that has come to be known as the man-eater. The white shark inhabits tropical and warm seas. Another species that will attack people is the tiger shark. Measuring up to 30 feet long, this shark is greatly feared in the West Indies and Australia. In 1988, I participated in the catching of a 28-foot, 3,000-pound tiger shark in the Pacific Ocean off the coast of Panama. Although it was an exhausting experience, no one suffered as a result of being attacked.

Around the world, fewer than 100 shark attacks are reported annually. Less than 30 of these are fatal. It has been determined that only 4 shark species—out of a total of at least 350 species—will attack humans. But it has also been said

that the only thing predictable about a shark is its unpre-
dictability. Whatever the actual number of attacks, these
incidents are still rare in relation to other calamities that can
befall us. Far more people die, for instance, of bee stings.
Sharks, after all, have better things to do than to look for
people to eat.

Because the shark is a predator, most of its energy is devoted to finding and consuming food. Its energy would, of
course, be better spent in eating than in chasing and capturing
its dinner. Sharks are, therefore, more likely to select weak or
dying prey. It is most often the blood from a fish speared by a
diver that attracts a shark. (Since the scent of blood often excites
a shark to attack, swimmers who might release blood into the
water—such as menstruating women—are advised to avoid
areas where sharks are found.)

Sometimes, a diver clad in a black wet suit and kicking his
flippers is mistaken for a seal, the shark's natural prey. If a
diver is attacked, the shark does not proceed beyond the first
bites. The diver is not the meal the shark wants. When fatalities
occur among divers or swimmers, they are more likely the
result of loss of blood than loss of body parts. Occasionally,
however, injured victims of air and sea disasters have been
eaten by hungry sharks on the prowl.

Now and then, a shark will attack a human whom it sees as
an invader of its territory. When a shark views a human as a
competitor, the attack is characterized by slashing wounds
with little tissue loss. These wounds are caused by the raking
motion of the upper jaw, which is obviously not a feeding
motion. A shark engaged in such aggressive behavior exhibits
definite signs—it shakes its head repeatedly and swims errati-
cally with its back hunched, pectoral fin down, and nose up.
The bloody damage depicted by the media is caused mostly by
a combination of the shark's biting action and the shaking of
its head. And, believe it or not, a shark's skin can also do great
damage to a diver.

SKIN

The skin of sharks is different from that of other fishes. Instead of scales, it has innumerable tiny "teeth" known as dermal denticles, or skin teeth. If you run your hand toward a shark's tail, the dermal denticles are pushed down and the skin feels smooth. But if you run your hand toward the nose and against the denticles, the skin is rough; in fact, it is so coarse that it can strip the skin off a swimmer with a sideways swipe of the shark's body.

Because of its texture, dried shark skin was once used as a sandpaper called shagreen. Today, shark hide is fashioned into a leather that is practically scuff-proof. This leather is used to make beautiful boots, shoes, and cases.

The skin of the shark is obviously not the only useful part of the animal. The oil contained in the shark's liver has also long had commercial uses.

LIVER

Sharks have enormous livers containing large amounts of oil that is very high in vitamin A. In fact, Borden's, one of the largest food companies in the United States, once operated a large shark-fishing division in Florida just to obtain the vitamin A in shark livers. During World War II, most of this important vitamin, so desperately needed for human and animal nutrition, was provided by Borden's. Before the war, it had come from sharks fished by the Japanese. Shortly after the war, vitamin A was synthesized by the Swiss, and the need for vitamin A obtained from natural shark liver oil was reduced to the point that the oil is now largely unused. This is a waste of an abundant resource.

The liver of a shark is so large that it constitutes as much as 25 percent of the shark's body weight. And because almost 100 percent of a shark's fat is stored in its liver, more than half of the weight of a shark liver is shark liver oil. This large liver and abundant oil supply are essential to the shark.

By storing lighter-than-water oil that decreases the density of the shark's body, the liver provides buoyancy. Many other species of fishes have an air bladder, a sac of gas that helps them swim and keeps them afloat when at rest. Sharks do not have this bladder, so they must swim or sink. The large oil-filled liver helps to keep them afloat. In addition, the liver is an energy store; all the fatty reserves are concentrated here. Because they can nourish themselves from the fat stores of these very large livers, sharks can survive even with only intermittent feedings. Sharks do, however, periodically engage in migrations that may be caused by the search for food.

MIGRATION

Generally speaking, sharks are warm-water creatures. They are found in a belt that circles the world at 20 degrees north to 20 degrees south of the equator (see Figure 1.2) and in warm-water currents like the Gulf Stream. However, although most sharks are found in warm salt waters, some live under the ice and others inhabit freshwater lakes and rivers. One ferocious freshwater species is found in Lake Nicaragua.

Daily migrations covering short distances are usually undertaken in pursuit of prey. Seasonal migrations that cover distances of unknown extent are often prompted by environmental factors such as temperature. Sharks are cold-blooded (poikilothermic); their body temperature conforms to that of the surrounding water. Shark species live in a temperature range determined by their metabolic or regulatory needs. Seasonal temperature changes cause species to migrate so that they can remain within the appropriate temperature range. Additional environmental factors that possibly cause sharks to mi-

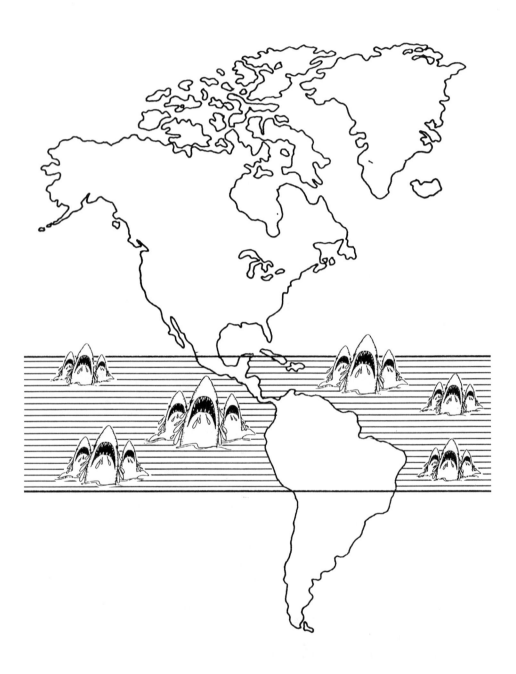

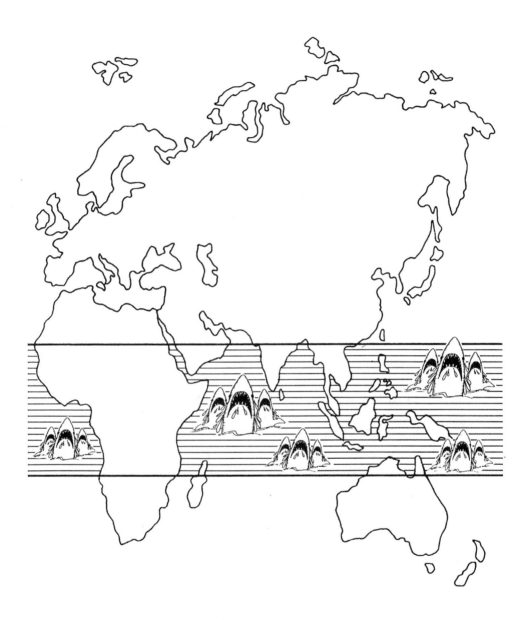

Figure 1.2. The shaded area on this world map shows the "belt" of heavy shark population.

grate include changes in oxygen solubility, light, and oceanic currents.

Other migrations of great distance are caused by mating habits. Some sharks travel to seemingly designated areas where they gather into large groups for mating purposes. Some of the females then migrate to specific areas, called nursery areas, where they give birth to the pups.

Migratory patterns reveal that sharks are segregated by sex but even more emphatically by size; a smaller shark always gives way to a larger. As one ichthyologist puts it, "The principal check on sharks is sharks themselves." In general, shark migration is poorly understood because it is difficult to track and study free-ranging sharks. Efforts to tag sharks and record their movements have not been very successful. Tagging has, however, garnered information about such attributes as the ages and sizes of sharks.

SIZES

Sharks come in a wide range of sizes. The most famous shark—or the most infamous, thanks to *Jaws*—is the white shark, which can be roughly as large as a city bus. One thirty-eight-foot white shark weighed in at thirteen tons, but white sharks can be twice as large as this behemoth. The largest shark ever caught was never weighed—there was no scale big enough. The smallest sharks can be held in the palm of your hand; one shark found in the Gulf of Mexico was only nine inches long.

REPRODUCTION

The smaller sharks lay eggs, but the larger species give birth to live young. Most cold-blooded creatures lay eggs. Typical fishes produce very large numbers of eggs and sperm, which are released into the water, where fertilization takes place.

After the young hatch, they require weeks or months to mature, meanwhile providing an easy meal for predators. The shark's success over the millenia is due at least in part to the adaptation of the external fertilization typical of bony fishes. Instead of being fertilized outside of the body, the eggs of most sharks are internally fertilized, and small numbers of large young are born live.

Another adaptation that has enhanced the shark's ability to reproduce and, therefore, to survive is the existence of two fully formed and operative male sex organs called claspers. While only one clasper is needed for reproduction at any one time, the shark is such a perfect survival machine that it is equipped with a spare should one clasper be lost in a fight or accident. During copulation, the male's clasper introduces sperm into the cloaca of the female.

All evidence indicates that copulation between sharks is strenuous if not downright dangerous. Partially healed cuts in pregnant females as well as firsthand observation in several aquariums reveal that males slash the females' pectoral fins and pelvic region to enlist cooperation in sexual activity. The wounds are not severe, and the females are able to engage in the nonstop swimming involved in copulation, which often lasts for more than a half-hour.

Following fertilization, there is a lengthy gestation period of about eleven months. Pups are usually born in the spring or early summer, either every year or every other year. With the larger, more commonly known shark species, an average brood consists of anywhere from twenty to eighty youngsters. These pups often measure two feet in length, weigh almost five pounds each, and are complete miniature replicas of their parents.

Being this large at birth assures the newborns a materially higher rate of survival than that of other cold-blooded offspring. The young of most fishes, though born in large numbers, have a very low survival rate. A newly hatched mackerel, for instance, measures one-eighth inch in length; twenty-six days later, it measures one-half inch. By the time it is forty days old, it has reached two inches in length and is the only survivor of a million mackerel spawned with it. The relatively large size and the capabilities of shark pups reduce the number of predators, and the percentage of surviving pups is large. However, the survival of the pups—and of the adults—also rests on the ability to resist disease.

SHARK IMMUNE SYSTEM

Sharks have a strong and very effective immune system. A shark's wounds heal rapidly, and sharks are largely free of infection. Antibodies contained in the blood successfully combat bacterial and viral infections as well as protect against a vast array of chemicals that easily kill most mammals.

Michael Sigel, chairman emeritus of the Department of Microbiology and Immunology at the University of South Carolina Medical School, was a pioneer in research on the immune system of the shark. In human beings, there are millions of possible antibodies, known as immunoglobulins, and the immune system is normally dormant, becoming active only in response to antigens. In the mid-1960s at the University of Miami, Sigel discovered that sharks have a peculiar immunoglobulin, a large amount of which is always circulating and ready to attack.

The shark's powerful immune system appears to produce antibodies against more than just bacteria, viruses, and chemicals, however. It also seems to help protect against cancer, whether the shark is bred and maintained in clean open waters or in carcinogen-laden enclosed waters (see page 43). This is the fact that gripped me back in the early 1980s and set me on a path full of questions about the why and how of the shark's resistance to cancer. What I especially wanted to know was how the information might be translated into a prevention or therapy for humans. I wanted to know just what sharks could do for us. It turns out that sharks have been doing a lot for people throughout time.

WHAT SHARKS CAN DO FOR PEOPLE

The shark has been on Earth for 400 million years; people (*Homo sapiens*) have been on Earth for some 500,000 years. In all the years that the two have lived together on this planet, people have found a myriad of ways in which the shark can make them healthier or more attractive.

For hundreds of years, people have hunted sharks for their hide, fins, oil, teeth, and meat. Tanned and with the denticles removed, good quality shark skin has twice the tensile strength of cowhide and has long been used to make a variety of leather goods. Fishermen used the skin as sandpaper, and the pattern on the surface of the skin was used by craftsmen to decorate a variety of objects such as inkstands, candlesticks, knives, and card cases. Shark teeth have long been used as jewelry as well as spear points and saws. The liver oil from the sand shark—abundant in the waters off Australia, where it is called the gray nurse—once lit the lamps of Sidney. But the principal use of sharks is food.

Shark meat is edible and highly regarded in some parts of the world. In Great Britain, for instance, the spurdog—which is sold as flake or rock salmon—accounts for a large portion of the fish used in fish and chips. Because all of a shark's oil is in its liver, the meat is dry and largely fat-free and tastes very much like swordfish.

Shark meat has not, however, enjoyed great popularity in North America, partially because the phrase "shark meat" has a negative connotation. The idea that sharks are "man-eaters" seems to render them singularly unappetizing. There has also been some fear that the shark's diet might cause its flesh to be toxic. Because sharks are scavengers, they accumulate heavy metals. These metals (for example, mercury, nickel, and copper)—referred to as "heavy" because they have a high molecular weight or high atomic number—are usually toxic in large quantities but in trace quantities may be important to health. While heavy metals are normally present in marginal amounts in shark meat, they are not present in the cartilage. Because the cartilage does not have any blood vessels, there is no way for the heavy metals to be carried into the cartilage. This is one reason why people in China have never suffered any toxic side effects from the shark-fin (a cartilage) soup they have eaten for generations.

Another reason shark meat is not popular in the United States is that it can have an ammonia-like smell if the blood is not drained directly after the fish is caught. Immediate salting or freezing should rectify this problem. Properly handled and prepared, boneless white shark steak is becoming popular on the West Coast, and there is even a recipe for it in the latest edition of the long-popular *Joy of Cooking*. It appears that the shark-fishing industry is beginning to burgeon.

Today's commercial shark fishing is carried out along the floors of the continental shelves (the slopes around the continents outside of which the ocean bed descends deeply), off large river mouths, and wherever a good food supply leads to abundant sea life. Sharks are often found with or near schools of tuna, where food is plentiful. Tuna fishermen catch many sharks, but they rarely harvest the meat since its commercial value has thus far been low. These fishermen want to use their refrigerated holding space for higher-priced tuna meat. When a shark is pulled aboard a tuna-fishing vessel, its fins are removed and sun-dried and its carcass is usually tossed back into the water. When the boats arrive in port, the crews sell the fins, which the Chinese use to make shark-fin soup. After long stints at sea, the crews use the money to finance onshore partying. Where shark is directly fished commercially, there is far less waste and less chance that wanton killing will endanger the species.

In those countries that have small fishing fleets engaged in purely local fishing—for instance, Mexico, Costa Rica, and other Central American countries; Cuba and other Caribbean nations; and many African nations—the entire shark is used. The meat is either salt-dried or eaten fresh, and the hides are often turned into leather. The fins, economically the most valuable part of the shark, are sold for use in soup. Shark-fin soup can be made from any or all of the shark's various fins—the dorsal fin, the lower tail fin, and the two pectoral, or large side, fins. A complete set of sun-dried fins from a shark weighing 150 pounds will sell for over $150. A wealthy Chinese gentleman will pay from $10 to $20 for a bowl of shark-fin soup.

Shark-fin soup has been eaten for countless years by the Chinese, usually daily and in large amounts. The Chinese have long recognized the health benefits of the cartilage in this soup. They consume shark cartilage in the belief that it is an aphrodisiac and an elixir of youth. Since the fibrous strands of cartilage are the desired part of shark-fin soup, this history of consumption is very sound evidence of shark cartilage's lack of toxicity and harmful side effects.

It is also interesting to note that the incidence of several forms of cancer (particularly breast cancer) is much lower in China than in the United States. Researchers agree that diet is one of the factors that accounts for the difference. The spaghetti-like protein fibers (see Figure 1.3) that are the main constituent of shark-fin soup are the same as those found in the shark's cartilaginous skeleton. These fibers, when properly processed as shark cartilage powder, give the amazing health benefits discussed in this book.

Healthful uses of shark products are not new. Up until the end of World War II, shark liver oil was, as discussed earlier in this chapter, the primary source of therapeutic vitamin A in the

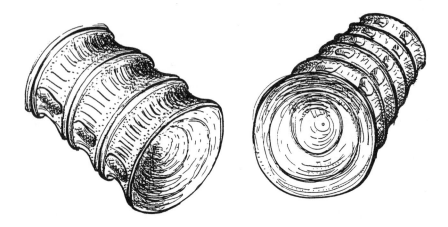

Figure 1.3. This drawing of a section of shark's backbone cartilage reveals the strands of protein and the matrix in which the protein fibers are imbedded.

world. In fact, shark liver oil yields ten times the amount of vitamin A found in the ever-unpopular cod liver oil. In 1939, at the height of shark-oil production, 9 million tons of sharks were caught for their oil. The industry was dead by 1950 after vitamin A was synthesized. In light of today's emphasis on natural products and conservation, perhaps shark liver oil can again become a common source of vitamin A.

Morton Walker, D.P.M., medical journalist, points out that sharks can supply more than vitamin A; he calls the shark a "floating nutritional factory." Dr. Walker says that in addition to vitamin A, the shark's liver is rich in a substance that Swedish scientist Astrid Brohult, M.D., claims will enhance healing in damaged human tissues. This substance also helps to build white blood cells, which is why one Norwegian physician believes that eating the white meat of a shark can be a defense against the harmful effects of radiation.

Sharks have also proven useful in the treatment of burn victims. In 1979 at Massachusetts General Hospital in Boston, a team led by John F. Burke, M.D., a surgeon and chief of trauma services, used shark cartilage to produce a successful human-skin substitute for the treatment of burns. An elementary principle of burn medicine is to remove from the body the skin destroyed by the burning heat. However, the exposed tissue, muscle, and fat must be covered at once. Dr. Burke was convinced that an artificial skin could be created to function like human skin without any rejection problems. Dr. Burke's efforts were aided by physical chemist Ioannis V. Yannas, a faculty member at MIT who has specialized in the study of collagen, a main constituent of both skin and cartilage.

Dr. Yannas knew that skin contains both collagen fibers and a complex structure called GAG (glycosaminoglycan). He believed that in the laboratory, collagen and GAG could be combined and chemically and physically treated to form a supple, porous material that would encourage the growth of healthy skin cells around it. GAG was extracted from shark cartilage and blended into a solution of collagen extracted from cowhide. The material was then freeze-dried, processed, shaped, and sterilized. Silicone adhesives were added to mimic the upper layer of human skin.

The substance was first tested in 1979 on an auto-accident victim who had burns covering nearly 60 percent of her body. The artificial skin was left in place for three weeks. When it was peeled away, there was a "quiltwork" of new tissue with blood vessels supplying it. Subsequent testing revealed that nerve endings had regenerated.

In addition to its use in artificial skin, shark cartilage in the form of capsules, powders, creams, suppositories, and injections has been in use since the early 1970s in therapy for inflammatory diseases. And many more healthful uses of shark cartilage may yet be discovered.

UTILIZATION RATHER THAN WASTE

Because of the many commercial uses for sharks, a great deal has been written about the possibility of overfishing. Actually, large numbers of sharks—an estimated 5 to 7 million—are already being caught each year. This figure is determined by calculating backwards based on the volume of dried shark fins annually imported into Hong Kong and Singapore and made into the popular shark-fin soup. This volume has been constant or growing modestly for at least fifteen years, suggesting a fairly healthy and abundant resource. There is certainly a need to prevent severe overfishing, but the real need is for greater utilization of the shark rather than waste of this valuable resource.

In resort areas in the United States such as Miami, Florida; Long Island, New York; and southern California, hundreds of sport fishermen yearly overfish sharks. These areas are usually in latitudes well beyond the equatorial belt in which the concentration of sharks is the greatest. Since sharks are often territorial, overfishing in an area remote from shark population centers can seriously deplete the population in that area. In addition, resorts in these areas have often reclaimed waterfront land, significantly reducing the wetlands and, therefore, the breeding capability of all sea life. Sharks, which live off of other sea life, are thus doubly hurt by resorts that prosper from sport fishing.

The shark population is also currently being depleted by some tuna fishermen and some fishermen who use large drift nets. Of the sharks caught for their fins by fishermen with the tuna fleet, approximately 95 percent are thrown away dead once the fins are removed, as just discussed. This squandering of meat and cartilage in an effort to harvest fins is a terrible waste of a most valuable resource, a resource that might be instrumental in preventing and curing some of man's worst diseases.

I know now that we can make use of sharks to improve our lives. This possibility is all the more exciting because it touches on diseases against which modern medicine has been largely ineffective. These are diseases for which the current therapeutic procedures are often quite devastating, producing side effects that are sometimes more destructive than the diseases themselves.

The exciting and remarkable shark has always fascinated people, largely because of our fear of and admiration for this supreme sea creature. Now, because of the significant health benefit discovered in shark cartilage, sharks are destined to play an increasingly important role in modern life.

2.

On the Trail

Scientists at the Massachusetts Institute of Technology have discovered a substance in shark cartilage that slows the growth of new blood vessels toward solid tumors, thereby cutting off tumor growth.

Warren E. Leary
Associated Press Science Writer

One reason sharks are so long-lived is they are one of the few living creatures that almost never get cancer. It now appears that the abundance of cartilage in sharks may explain why these fish are not prone to cancer and may give man a way to prevent and cure this most devastating disease. But the knowledge did not come overnight. Instead, it evolved slowly, in bits and pieces, like a detective story.

In the manner of detectives, scientists pile clue upon clue, pursuing a trail until all the information is in and the mystery is solved. But in science, the detective work is called research and the trail begins with a hypothesis, an idea to be proven or disproven. The clues are rarely uncovered in drawing rooms where butlers serve sherry. They result instead from experiments and case studies that may eventually lead to "solving the mystery" and controlling a dreaded disease.

THE TRAIL BEGINS

In the United States, one of the earliest experiments aimed at controlling cancer involved a factor in cells that could cause the death (necrosis) of a tumor. Now called the tumor necrosis factor (TNF), its existence had been suspected since William B. Coley, M.D., a researcher and a surgeon at Memorial Hospital in New York City from 1892 to 1931, experimented with a new therapy in the 1890s. Coley's treatment of cancer patients with a vaccine made from mixed killed bacteria sometimes resulted in tumor regression. Years later, other researchers working with mice found that Coley's vaccine caused tumors to bleed into themselves, turn black, and dry up, a process called hemorrhagic necrosis. Subsequent testing of the vaccine showed it would not kill tumors that were being kept alive in test tubes, a finding that led to a search for anticancer forces within a living organism that might be stimulated by bacterial products. In the 1970s, this force—tumor necrosis factor—was identified and later shown to damage the blood vessels that nourish tumors. This damage to the blood vessels reduces the flow of blood and oxygen to the tumor cells, which then starve and die.

Once the action of tumor necrosis factor—namely, a diminished supply of blood and oxygen—was identified, it remained for researchers to determine how best to cut off this supply. The hypothesis of one New England investigator working three decades after the death of Dr. Coley was to set other investigators on the path that led to the discovery discussed in this book. And how perfect it is that an area famous for its fishing industry would unknowingly spawn a theory whose success would depend on a fish!

TUMOR GROWTH IN VITRO PROVIDES A CLUE

In the 1960s in Boston, Massachusetts—home of scrod and lobster—Judah Folkman, M.D., of Children's Hospital and Harvard Medical School, was working on a hypothesis about the nature of tumors. A tumor is new tissue made of cells that grow in an uncontrolled manner. In normal tissue, growth is limited; the rate of cell reproduction is equal to the rate of cell death. Tumors can be benign or malignant. Benign tumors are rarely fatal, although they may interfere with the body's normal functions. Malignant tumors proliferate and invade surrounding normal tissues, eventually metastasizing (spreading to other places within the body) via the blood vessels and lymph system. It is this runaway duplication of cancer cells that makes them so life-threatening—a growing tumor mass will eventually suffocate vital organs, starving them of nutrients and other resources. When the vital organs die, so does the host. Preventing cancer and/or cancer fatalities might then depend on stopping the runaway duplication of cells.

Like all investigators of the time, Dr. Folkman knew that tumors have—and require—a rich blood supply to feed their growth. During his studies with animals, Dr. Folkman noted that tumors implanted in isolated organs—organs maintained outside the body *in vitro* (in artificial environments)—grew to only a few millimeters in diameter. The same tumors implanted in mice grew rapidly, eventually killing the mice. What was the difference between an organ maintained in a liquid medium and an organ functioning in a living organism? In the living organisms—the mice—the tumors developed a blood network; in the liquid medium, they did not. It took several more years before the significance of this discovery was fully understood.

Researchers eventually came to realize that in isolated organs, the capillary endothelium—the layer of cells lining the capillaries—degenerates rapidly, causing the death of the capillaries. Without tiny blood vessels to nourish them, tumors cannot grow.

Then, in 1971, Dr. Folkman published his now-famous hypothesis in *The New England Journal of Medicine*. His main points were:

- Tumors cannot grow without a network of blood vessels to nourish them and to remove waste products.

- Inhibiting the development of blood vessels could be a potential cancer therapy.

Dr. Folkman's theory sounds simple enough. But it was like a key without a lock. It took almost twenty years for the theory to be used to open doors leading to disease control. One of the first steps on the twenty-year path was to understand the process that Dr. Folkman had hypothesized, a process that came to be known as *antiangiogenesis.*

The term *angiogenesis* was coined in 1935 to describe the formation of new blood vessels in the placenta during pregnancy. It comes from the Greek words *angio*, meaning "blood," and *genesis*, meaning "formation of." As used today, angiogenesis refers to the formation of new blood vessels during an individual's development or growth, or to the replacement of injured vessels in existing tissue.

In a normal adult, the blood network is well established. Angiogenesis occurs only infrequently—during ovulation and pregnancy, in the healing of wounds and fractures, and in certain heart and/or circulatory conditions. The only other time angiogenesis—also called *neovascularization*—seems to occur is during the development of a tumor or other malady associated with the need for a new blood network. Adding these facts together, Dr. Folkman felt that if angiogenesis could be stopped, tumor growth could be stopped. Without a network of blood vessels to supply it with nutrients and to remove waste materials, a tumor would simply die. Without nourishment, there can be no growth; it's that simple. But where could inhibitors be found or how could they be developed?

Researchers decided to look for an angiogenesis inhibitor in cartilage. They reasoned that since cartilage is avascular (without blood vessels), it might have a way of keeping the blood vessels from developing. (See "Why Cartilage Is Antiangiogenic" on page 42.) According to Patricia D'Amore, Ph.D., of the Laboratory of Surgical Research, Children's Hospital, Boston, "The rationale for the use of avascular tissue extracts is that these tissues are devoid of vessels because they contain inhibitors of angiogenesis."

Blood vessels appear in cartilage only as a preliminary to bone formation during the fetal stage or to the calcification that occurs in arthritic conditions. At these times, cartilage's ability to inhibit angiogenesis seems to loose its efficacy.

FINDING AN ANGIOGENESIS INHIBITOR

In 1973, researchers at Rush-Presbyterian-St. Luke's Medical Center in Chicago implanted small pieces of cartilage into the fetal membrane of a chick embryo. This membrane is called the chorioallantoic membrane. The researchers observed that the cartilage was not invaded by blood vessels although vessels did invade other implanted tissues.

Beginning in the mid-1970s, another team of scientists, this one working at the Massachusetts Institute of Technology (MIT), was also considering the inhibition of vascularization. Robert Langer, Sc.D., and Anne Lee, Ph.D., reported in the prestigious journal *Science* that the cartilage found in the shoulders of calves could inhibit the vascularization of solid tumors. In their experiment, Langer and Lee infused an extract of cartilage from the shoulders of calves into rabbits and mice.

Why Cartilage Is Antiangiogenic

In recent years, observation of chick embryos has given scientists a great deal of information about the development and special properties of cartilage. The scientists noted that in chick embryos, the limb "bud" is nourished by capillaries. One of the capillaries near the center of the limb soon becomes enlarged and forms the major limb artery. Near this artery, in the core of the limb, the remaining capillaries disappear. By the fourth day of the embryo's development (half a day before limb cells become committed to particular developmental paths), no capillaries remain in the core of the limb. At the edge of the limb, the major artery becomes a complex capillary bed.

The cells at the very center of the limb probably produce a substance that inhibits vascularization. These cells eventually develop into cartilage. The substance that inhibits vascularization appears to be present in cartilage throughout the life of the tissue and is probably the reason why cartilage is antiangiogenic.

Although the animals exhibited no signs of toxicity, the growth of new blood vessels toward implanted tumors ceased and tumor growth stopped.

The research at MIT should have advanced the search for an angiogenesis inhibitor quite rapidly, but further research was thwarted. Drs. Langer and Lee claimed that this was caused by the short supply of the cartilage extract, due to mammals' having only a small amount of cartilage. These researchers decided, therefore, to turn to sharks, whose skeletons are composed entirely of cartilage. Their decision was not entirely unprecedented. Carl Luer, Ph.D., a biochemist at Mote Marine Laboratory in Sarasota, Florida, was already doing research involving sharks and disease. His research was based on a fact that had been well known for almost a dozen years—sharks rarely develop cancer, either naturally or when exposed to massive amounts of highly carcinogenic chemicals.

SHARKS RESIST TUMORS NATURALLY

When Dr. Luer exposed sharks to high levels of aflatoxin B_1, a substance that is considered very carcinogenic, the sharks did not display an elevated incidence of tumors. Aflatoxin B_1 is actually a precursor of a carcinogen. When aflatoxin is activated, the resulting product bonds with DNA and probably attacks genes that would otherwise prevent the expression of cancer by cells. Aflatoxin is activated in the liver through the action of certain enzymes. Dr. Luer and his associates from Clemson University found that shark livers have only 20 percent of a calf liver's ability to activate aflatoxin B_1. The implication is that sharks may be only 20 percent as likely as calves to develop cancer. This would seem to be consistent with the lower incidence of tumors in sharks. In other words, sharks may be only 20 percent as likely as calves to develop cancer under the same conditions.

Dr. Luer is currently conducting experiments to determine why sharks resist cancer. He gets cartilage from bull and sandbar sharks in the waters off Florida. Testing of protein extracts from the cartilage has indicated that there are six or seven proteins that have the ability to prevent blood-vessel growth.

SHARK CARTILAGE IS COMPARED
WITH BOVINE CARTILAGE

Armed with the same knowledge about sharks as Dr. Luer, Dr. Langer and Dr. Lee began their second study on antiangiogenesis by preparing an extract of shark cartilage containing the purest possible form of the angiogenesis inhibitor. This extract was placed in polymer-type pellets, and the pellets were implanted in pockets behind the corneas of New Zealand white rabbits. A virulent strain of carcinoma was then implanted behind the pellets. Control animals were also implanted with tumors and pellets, but these latter pellets did not contain the shark-cartilage extract.

Drs. Langer and Lee saw that the tumor implants caused blood vessels to grow toward them from the rim of the cornea. Using sophisticated microscopy techniques, the researchers measured the length of the longest vessels. In three separate studies, they found that the extract inhibited angiogenesis. All of the control (untreated) animals had large three-dimensional tumors with blood vessels averaging a maximum length of 6 millimeters. Animals that had received the cartilage implant had neither three-dimensional tumors nor any vascularization around the pellets. In these treated corneas, the average maximum length of blood vessels was 1.5 millimeters, 75 percent shorter than the average maximum length in the control animals.

These studies lasted only nineteen days. Tumor growth began on day fourteen, when the blood network was in place. Once they could receive nutrients, the tumors grew dramatically in only five days.

The study had a second outcome that would—eventually—bring the shark to the forefront of angiogenesis research. It was discovered that shark-cartilage extracts require far less purification than do bovine-cartilage extracts to achieve inhibition of angiogenesis. Because there is so little fat clinging to shark cartilage as compared with bovine cartilage, the shark cartilage can be said to be "purer" to begin with. Therefore, while 1 milligram of cancer-inhibiting extract can be recovered from 500 grams of calf cartilage, Langer and Lee report that the same amount of inhibitor can be processed from only 0.5 gram of shark cartilage. In other words, 500 grams of calf cartilage is needed to produce 1 milligram of a substance that can inhibit vascular growth by 70 percent. This is less inhibition than was achieved with one-thousandth as much material derived from a shark, which means shark cartilage, on a pound-for-pound basis, is *1,000 times* more potent as a cancer inhibitor than is cartilage obtained from cows and other mammals. In addition, the amount of cartilage in an average shark far exceeds the amount of cartilage in an average calf.

PROVING THE MEDICAL POTENTIAL OF CARTILAGE

Although Langer and Lee had proven the efficacy of shark cartilage as an inhibitor of angiogenesis, their research seemed to languish. As a matter of fact, a major clinical study published *two years later* dealt with the treatment of cancer using bovine-cartilage extracts. This study was published in 1985 by Harvard-trained surgeon John Prudden, M.D., Med.Sc.D., an early pioneer in the use of cartilage to accelerate wound healing.

Despite the evidence presented by the studies at MIT—studies that Dr. Prudden lists as references in his own publication—Dr. Prudden continued to pursue bovine research. His work is of major import because he established the validity of using cartilage of any kind in medical applications. His earlier studies with cartilage had shown beneficial wound-healing effects when cartilage powder derived from a variety of sources was applied as a topical preparation. It is interesting to note that *today's* surgical texts routinely include discussions of how animal-cartilage preparations can be used to accelerate wound healing, a treatment that Dr. Prudden experimented with in 1960. The inclusion of this information in the texts is quite a shift in traditional medicine because authorities had always held that wound-healing in a healthy animal, an animal whose endocrine system was normal and who was nutritionally sound, would occur at a certain speed regardless of the use of any wound-healing accelerators. The acceptance of the belief that a cartilage preparation can speed up healing in even a healthy animal should make it easier for the traditional medical community to accept the other properties of cartilage preparations.

Dr. Prudden's cancer study is also very exciting because it was the first time that cancer patients were successfully treated using cartilage as an immune-system stimulator and mild angiogenesis inhibitor. Just imagine—when cancer patients were given bovine cartilage, their tumors shrank, and *shark cartilage is reputed to be 1,000 times more effective as an angiogenesis inhibitor.* In addition, shark cartilage has the same capability of stimulating the immune system as does bovine cartilage.

In Dr. Prudden's study, thirty-one patients with a variety of cancers and tumors were treated. Dr. Prudden reported a major inhibitory effect using oral and injected bovine cartilage. Patient response was measured over an eleven-year period to gauge the long-term success of the treatment.

Dr. Prudden had begun the study in 1972 with patients for whom it was believed standard radiation and chemotherapy would be of no value. The patients' rate of survival improved when they received the calf cartilage, which was first injected and then orally administered. The injection phase was called the loading phase. Two to four injections were given per visit for a total dose of 100 milliliters per treatment, repeated from once a week up to every other day. The loading phase concluded when 2,000 milliliters had been injected, at which time oral dosage began. The oral phase was the maintenance phase. Eight capsules, each containing 375 milligrams of the powdered cartilage, were administered every eight hours. There was no evidence that a dosing schedule was critical, providing that at least 9 grams of the cartilage were taken per day in at least two doses.

There was also no evidence of any toxicity; no abnormalities were ever reported in tests of kidney or liver function or in blood values. All toxicity testing as required by the Food and Drug Administration (FDA) proved negative, including a two-year carcinogenesis study and a sixteen-month study to determine if physical defects were produced in offspring (teratogenicity study). The results of the experiment presented a fantastic picture—Dr. Prudden reported tumor regression without the debilitating effects of chemotherapy, radiation, or surgery.

In evaluating his results, Dr. Prudden considered that a patient had a "complete response" when all clinical evidence of an active tumor had disappeared for a minimum of twelve weeks. A skeletal radiograph (an image showing where a radioactive substance is concentrated) must have clearly shown improvement, with all injuries or abnormalities (lesions) exhibiting evidence of renewed bone growth. A 50-percent decrease in the size of measured lesions or in any pretreatment tumor markers (substances in the body linked to a cancer) was considered a partial response. There could be no simultaneous increase in the size of any lesions or markers or an appearance of new lesions or markers; the response had to have been maintained for at least twelve weeks. A patient was considered to have had minimal response if there was a decrease in tumor size of less than 50 percent but more than 25 percent along with a 25- to 50-percent reduction in tumor markers, significant improvement in bone pain, and significant improvement in clinical neurological examination in cases of brain cancer. An increase of at least 25 percent in the size of any measured lesion or tumor marker or the appearance of any new lesion or marker was considered progression of disease. Relapse was defined as the appearance of new lesions, the reappearance of old lesions in patients who had achieved a complete response, or an increase of 50 percent or more in the sum of measurable tumor mass in patients who had achieved partial response.

Using the above criteria, Dr. Prudden concluded that cartilage had a "major inhibitory effect upon a wide spectrum of cancers." A complete response with probable or possible cure was noted in eleven of the thirty-one cases (35 percent). The eleven cases included:

- A patient with uterine cervix cancer who at the time Dr. Prudden's paper was published had gone more than seven years without a recurrence of the disease.

- A patient with pancreatic carcinoma who had gone eight years without a recurrence.

- A patient with squamous cell cancer of the nose who had gone five years without a recurrence.

Complete response with relapse was documented in 26 percent of the cases, and a partial response, in 19 percent. A total of 3 percent of the patients displayed no change, and 3 percent showed disease progression. Dr. Prudden's conclusion, printed in the *Journal of Biological Response Modifiers*, was, "When confronted by entities such as pancreatic cancer, squamous or adenocarcinoma of the lung, glioblastoma multiforme, and other situations where present therapeutic impotence is clear, the use of Catrix [powdered calf cartilage] therapy as the primary agent should be considered. One persuasive argument for using it in this way is that, in happy contrast to chemotherapy, it burns no immunological or hematological bridges."

There are no words that express how excited I was to learn of Dr. Prudden's work. But I was—and am still—amazed that the work did not inspire a line-up of people trying to realize the potential of cartilage as a cancer therapy. To my knowledge, there has still been little or no follow-up of Dr. Prudden's study. One of the few scientists who pursued similar research was Dr.

Brian G. M. Durie of the Department of Internal Medicine at the University of Arizona Health Sciences Center. Dr. Durie conducted research into the antitumor effects of bovine cartilage the same year Dr. Prudden undertook his work. A paper by Dr. Durie states that when bovine cartilage was applied directly to tumor cells maintained in a test tube or other artificial environment, practically all of the tumor cells were killed. Using three human-tumor cell lines (cell tissue cultures parented by three specific types of human tumor cells) and fresh biopsy specimens from twenty-two patients with malignant tumors, Dr. Durie was able to demonstrate efficacy against ovarian, pancreatic, colon, testicular, and sarcoma biopsy specimens with continuous high-dose exposure to Catrix. Perhaps the most significant sensitivity was seen in the ovarian cancer samples. This is particularly important since almost half of all ovarian cancers are considered inoperable. Dr. Durie concluded that the results with the crude cartilage extracts justified additional in vitro evaluation and consideration of expanded clinical trials. But no one conducted these trials. Can it be that nothing turns more slowly than the wheels of the medical establishment?

The wheels seem to be turning with excruciating slowness when one considers that almost two decades after Dr. Folkman's initial hypothesis, another New England investigator began claiming that angiogenesis inhibitors not only stop tumor growth but also prevent the spread of metastases.

ANGIOGENESIS INHIBITION PREVENTS METASTASIS

According to an article published in 1988 by Dr. Patricia D'Amore, "The only event that stands between maintenance of metastatic cells in a dormant state and their establishment into a secondary tumor is the development of a vasculature [system of blood vesssels]. Thus, therapies aimed at interfering with vascularization represent viable strategies for antimetastasis."

Dr. D'Amore expressed the belief that vascularization is "clearly essential for the establishment and subsequent growth of metastases." She also believed that inhibition of angiogenesis may be a way of preventing metastasis. This concept would be conclusively proven one year later by a team of Boston physicians that included Dr. Folkman (see page 52).

Meanwhile, Dr. Prudden, one of the earliest "detectives" in the case, had not disappeared from the scene. He was conducting experiments into the immunoregulatory effects of cartilage. His research revealed that Catrix-S, an injectable form of Catrix, enhanced antibody production. The complex carbohydrates in cartilage known as mucopolysaccharides apparently give cartilage other therapeutic benefits besides angiogenesis inhibition. It is the mucopolysaccharides that have the immunoregulatory effect, and they also have an anti-inflammatory effect. The mucopolysaccharides chondroitin sulfate A and C have long been known to fight inflammation. It now seemed that the naturally occurring form of these compounds in shark cartilage was more effective than synthetically refined mucopolysaccharides. However, this level of effectiveness combined with the antiangiogenesis and immunoregulatory effects in whole cartilage still did not seem to present researchers with sufficient reason to experiment with whole natural cartilage. Instead, Dr. Langer remained hard at work with his extracts of cartilage.

In 1990, Langer and his associates published a paper in *Science* in which they reported that they had identified as a strong angiogenesis inhibitor a specific macromolecule derived from cartilage. The scientists appeared to be trying to isolate a particular protein found in cartilage that would work as an inhibitor of angiogenesis. This inhibitor, as we have seen, would have the potential of stopping tumor growth and preventing metastasis. At this point, Langer and his associates were still seeking the best possible inhibitor, proving, according to the *Science* article, that the potency of the angiogenesis inhibitor increased with increasing purification.

Dr. Langer and his associates were able to graphically demonstrate that an extract of bovine cartilage could prevent neovascularization in living organisms. Their experiments involved microscopic investigations of fertilized chick embryos. These embryos were placed in petri dishes, and the cartilage extract was applied to the surfaces of the embryos. In repeated tests, microscopic analysis revealed that there were areas in the embryos where vascularization was being inhibited (see Figure 2.1). This testing process, called the chick chorioallantoic membrane, or CAM, assay led the scientists to conclude that the study might explain why some tissues are resistant to invasion by capillary cells and might help them understand how to control blood-vessel growth.

Also in 1990, a publication by Japanese researchers reported a crude separation of a second and possibly a third protein in shark cartilage responsible for the inhibition of angiogenesis. These proteins are different from the ones that were reported by Langer. It thus appears that natural whole shark cartilage probably has at least two, and possibly more, independent inhibitors of angiogenesis.

WHY WONDER WHY?

I understand that scientists are perfectionists and that theories must be tested and tested again in order to be proven conclusively. Yet, I cannot help but wonder about the emphasis on determining exactly *what* it is in tissues such as cartilage that resists neovascularization. When human lives are at stake, isn't it enough to know that the tissues *do* resist invasion and therefore resist the formation of tumors and metastases? Isn't it enough to know that shark cartilage is a naturally occurring product that has been eaten by people for countless genera-

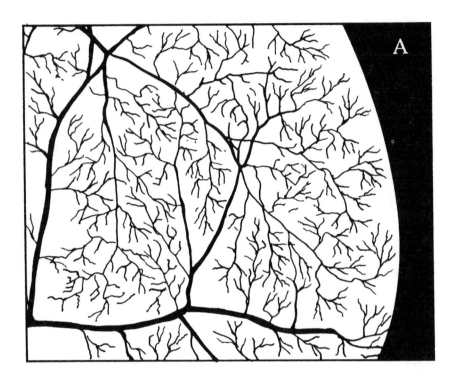

Figure 2.1. These pictures of fertilized chicken eggs show capillary growth in normal circumstances and after the implantation of a pellet containing shark cartilage. Drawing A depicts the microscopic field of capillaries growing into the fertilized yolk sac of a chicken egg under regular conditions. Drawing B shows the microscopic field

tions? Why would it take another half-dozen years before shark cartilage would be tested on victims of one of the most debilitating diseases known to man, a disease so dreaded that there are people who will not even say the word "cancer"?

Instead of leading to clinical trials, the research path led to a study, reported in *The New England Journal of Medicine* on January 3, 1991, proving Dr. D'Amore's belief that without vascularization, there is little metastasis. The study was conducted by a team of four physicians led by Noel Weidner, M.D., and including Dr. Folkman. Experimentation with mi-

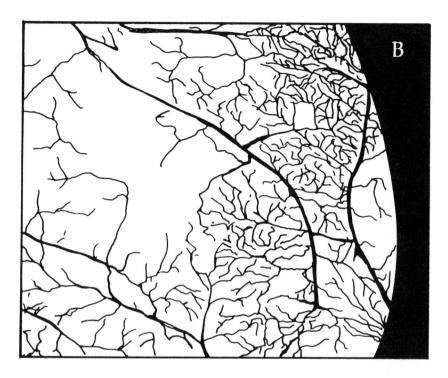

of capillaries growing in a chick embryo after a pellet containing shark cartilage was implanted. The cartilage is having an antiangiogenic effect where the pellet was implanted (in the area in the left half of drawing B), resulting in the growth of fewer capillaries.

croscopically viewed zones of vascularization gave strong evidence that metastasis is as angiogenesis-dependent as are tumors. The researchers reported in *The New England Journal of Medicine*, "The amount of neovascularization measured directly in histologic [diseased cell] sections of breast carcinoma correlates with the presence of metastasis, and this information may prove useful even before we understand why it is true."

Experimental evidence proved that there is a prevascular phase as well as a vascular phase in the development of carcinomas of the cervix, bladder, and breast. The limited tumor growth during the prevascular stage is followed by the rapid tumor growth, bleeding, and potential metastasis that characterizes the vascular phase. The physicians further demonstrated that lesions having little vascularization have a much lower rate of metastasis than lesions having advanced angiogenesis. This evidence is particularly important in cases of breast tumors because, as had been previously demonstrated by researchers, breast cancer begins to metastasize when the tumors are quite small. Even early detection procedures may be too late to prevent metastasis, the real killer. (Radiologists reading mammograms, for instance, cannot detect tumors smaller than one-half inch unless the tumors are dense.) Such evidence means that shark cartilage's potential of halting vascularization and therefore stopping metastasis may be truly vital to the prevention of breast cancer.

Weidner's study, which involved forty-nine women with breast cancer—thirty patients with metastases and nineteen without—also showed the correlation between vascularization and tumor metastasis. By counting the number of capillaries and venules (small blood vessels that collect blood from the capillaries) in a microscopic field of excised tumor tissue, the researchers were able to demonstrate that angiogenesis correlates with metastasis in breast carcinoma. In addition, they determined that the density of microvessels (capillaries and venules) correlates with the development of metastatic disease. In other words, the chances of metastasis increase as the vessel count increases. With up to thirty-three blood vessels in a 200X field, the chances of metastasis are only 14 percent; with thirty-four to sixty-seven blood vessels per microscopic field, the chances are 45 percent; with sixty-eight to one hundred blood vessels per microscopic field, the chances are 71 percent; with over one hundred blood vessels per microscopic field, the chances are 100 percent.

The same researchers also graded the density of the capillaries and venules in the breast carcinomas. It was shown that for each ten-vessel increase in the microvessel count, there was a 1.17-fold increase in the risk of distant metastasis.

Weidner and his colleagues concluded that there is a "significant correlation between the density of microvessels in histologic sections of invasive breast carcinoma . . . and the occurrence of metastases." They also wrote, "For a tumor cell to metastasize . . . tumor cells must gain access to the vasculature from the primary tumor, survive travel through the circulation, settle in the microvasculature into the target organ, and induce angiogenesis in the target organ."

It is easier for tumor cells to penetrate newly developing capillaries than mature vessels. Angiogenesis therefore provides a perfect route for tumor cells to move into the circulatory system, causing metastasis. In addition, the tumor cells at the metastatic site must induce angiogenesis if they are to survive. This is more likely to occur when the primary tumor is highly angiogenic.

A TRAIL DECADES OLD

With the dawn of the 1990s, more than twenty years had passed since the relationship between tumor growth and angiogenesis had been first postulated. And what did we have? Proof positive that:

- Both tumor growth and the spread of metastasis require the development of a new blood network.

- Development of a new blood network can be inhibited by the use of an extract of shark cartilage.

Yet, researchers were still ignoring the therapeutic and prophylactic potentials of shark cartilage. In 1991, Dr. Folkman investigated a variety of other angiogenesis inhibitors that might be used as therapeutic and preventative tools. In the book *Biologic Therapy of Cancer*, he discusses thirteen substances that inhibit angiogenesis.

One of the substances Dr. Folkman discusses is, like shark cartilage, a naturally occurring substance that he has used to inhibit angiogenesis. Heparin, a mucopolysaccharide acid occurring in several tissues but most abundantly in the liver and lungs, has been used for years as an intravenous injection that prevents blood from clotting. It is therefore useful in the prevention and treatment of thrombosis (a condition in which a blood clot develops within a blood vessel) and postoperative pulmonary embolism (a condition in which a lung artery is blocked by foreign matter), and in the repair of vascular injury. However, the same anticoagulant property of heparin that is so useful also makes it unsafe to use as an angiogenesis inhibitor for an extended period of time.

Another difficulty in using heparin therapeutically is that its ability to bring about angiogenesis is variable. Both this variability and the difficult process involved in synthesizing even a small amount of heparin have stimulated a search for substitutes. Many of the possibilities have proven to be toxic, and the effectiveness of some seems to be limited to specific situations. Tests were therefore run on substances that could be combined with heparin to neutralize its anticoagulant activity and leave its ability to inhibit angiogenesis intact or even enhanced.

Of the thirteen substances tested by Dr. Folkman and reviewed in *Biologic Therapy of Cancer,* all—except for cartilage—displayed some level of toxicity and could not be used over an extended period. The use of angiogenesis inhibition as a preventive necessitates long-term administration, so the toxicity level must be very low or nonexistent in the administered inhibitor. Whether antiangiogenic therapy is used alone or in conjunction with conventional chemotherapy, Dr. Folkman writes in the above book, "It is clear that angiogenesis inhibitors . . . may need to be administered for prolonged periods. Such long-term therapy will require compounds of relatively low toxicity."

Both the toxicity of many angiogenesis inhibitors and the difficulty of synthesizing them make the use of a natural product such as shark cartilage very attractive. Heparin-steroid combinations, however, are useful as the standard by which angiogenesis inhibition can be measured. (See "Measuring Angiogenesis-Inhibiting Activity" on page 58.)

On the CAM assay, the scale derived for evaluation, hydrocortisone-heparin receives an index of 0.55 to 0.75. Pure shark-cartilage powder refined so that it contains at least 39 percent protein and less than 0.4 percent fat receives a minimum CAM assay index of 0.85, varying up to 1.1 on the high side. The potency of shark cartilage as an angiogenesis inhibitor increases with its increasing protein content.

LOOKING AT THE EVIDENCE

Respected researchers from prestigious institutions had for decades been piling up clues in the fight against cancer. The evidence they had amassed presented a most promising picture. Consider:

- Few, if any, sharks get cancer.

- Tumors and metastases cannot develop without a network of blood vessels to support them.

- Tumor growth is dependent upon the growth of new blood vessels.

- Growth of new blood vessels (angiogenesis) does not normally occur in adults.

- Cartilage has no blood vessels.

- Shark's skeletons are composed primarily of cartilage.

- Shark cartilage is the most effective nontoxic substance for prohibiting angiogenesis. (The antiangiogenesis effect, it is

Measuring Angiogenesis-Inhibiting Activity

Measuring angiogenesis-inhibiting activity enables us to judge and compare products and standardize their effectiveness. A technique called the chicken chorioallantoic membrane (CAM) assay is used to measure how a test product affects vascularization in a membrane of a newly fertilized and incubated chicken embryo (see Figure 2.1 on pages 52–53).

A pellet containing the material to be tested is placed directly on the developing vessels in the chick embryo. The development or inhibition of new vessels is then measured. After the extent of new vascularization is determined, the test product is given a numerical rating, called the vascularization index (VI). A score of 2.0 is perfect, and 0 (zero) reflects no effect. A CAM activity range of 0.85 to 1.1 is considered effective angiogenesis inhibition.

Test products are often compared with a combination of heparin and cortisone formulated by Dr. Judah Folkman. When batches of shark cartilage were tested, they were found to be equal in effectiveness to the heparin-cortisone standard. As processing techniques improved, shark cartilage was shown to materially exceed the heparin-cortisone standard. The vascularization index as well as the size of the area of reduced vascularity generally surpassed the standard. Recent developments in extraction techniques are yielding a shark-cartilage product that has a higher concentration of protein and will, therefore, get even higher CAM assay figures.

Consumers can be assured of the efficacy of a product through the use of the vascularization index. Properly utilized, this important tool can ensure that only high-quality shark-cartilage products are offered to the public.

now clear, is shark cartilage's main weapon, a weapon that works synergistically with the mucopolysaccharides.)

Although these clues had been piling up for over twenty years, researchers were not taking the final step to solving the mystery. There were no tests of shark cartilage's ability to cure cancer in humans. After I literally stumbled across the information scientists had been privy to for so long, I marshalled whatever resources I could to move the studies forward.

3.

Putting Theory
Into Action

*... antiangiogenic therapy could restrict the
growth of a wide variety of solid tumors while
being administered for prolonged periods, with
low toxicity and a low probability of drug
resistance.*

M. Judah Folkman, M.D.
Harvard Medical School
Biologic Therapy of Cancer

Although the scientific detectives knew that they were on to something, their training had them conditioned to look for a pure chemical that could be isolated, synthesized, and patented. This is the way the research game is played in this country. The only way a company can make a "breakthrough" is to get FDA approval for a drug so that it can get a patent, protect itself against competition, advertise, and recoup the approximately $231 million spent doing the testing required by the FDA. When I found out about the potential for a cancer cure—a potential that was languishing—I was amazed, excited, and appalled all at once and decided to do something about it. While the researchers tested, analyzed, and retested in their laboratories, I went out in the field, where my background enabled me to accomplish things that researchers cannot find the time to do. Although I have had an extensive scientific education and many years in research, I am also an experienced international businessman.

A DIFFERENT EYE ON THE CASE

Because I went to college during the Depression, I attended the School of Agriculture at Cornell University, which was free. At that time, Cornell's School of Agriculture was quite the place to learn about farming and the agricultural industry. It also had an extensive course offering in nutrition. While most colleges during the 1930s may have had only a few, if any, courses on nutrition, Cornell offered enough variety and depth for a student to major in the field. And the more I learned about nutrition, the more interested in it I became—so interested, in fact, that I went on to receive a master's in nutritional science from Cornell and a doctorate in agricultural biochemistry and nutrition from Rutgers University.

My solid background and continued interest in the field are the result of the quality of my instructors. I was fortunate enough to study under several distinguished nutritional pioneers, including two future Nobel Prize winners—Dr. James B. Sumner, who won the prize for chemistry in 1946, and Dr. Selman Waksman, who won the prize for physiology and medicine in 1952.

By the time I finished my education and my army service, the field of nutritional science was really coming into its own. I found a research position in the feed industry in which I came up with the idea of premixing and packaging nutritional supplements to be added to animal feed. In this way, feed manufacturers could have a custom mix that would be used to make specific animal and poultry feeds. Later on, I became involved in the use of fishmeal as a feed additive.

The United States fishmeal industry had been dominated by one family, which owned 60 percent of the production capability of the industry. When Peru entered the business, the supply of fishmeal doubled and prices plummeted, making the business an economic nightmare. But I thought things could be salvaged. I said, "The business can't fall any further. The only way it can go is up. Let's try increasing the percentage of fishmeal in chicken feed." As the percentage of fishmeal was increased, the chickens fared better, and the fishmeal market boomed once again.

The boom kept me busy traveling all over the country in my capacity as president of the Fishmeal Trade Association and as a leader of symposia about the advantages of fishmeal in feed until representatives of W. R. Grace and Company recruited me as a vice president for the new Marine Resources Division. It was in this position that I learned how to buy and sell companies, how to fund projects, how to be a man of action more than theory. I guess I learned my lessons well because President Ronald Reagan soon called upon me to serve on a presidential mission assisting the West African country of Guinea. That newly emerging nation, first having turned leftist and then rightist, was attempting to establish a place for itself in the world market. Its leaders had identified its key resources—fishing, agriculture, and aluminum—and President Reagan was now sending an expert in each of the resource areas to identify investment opportunities. My practical eye was able to discern big opportunities for the fishing industry, and I was subsequently called upon to speak to the United States Department of State about getting things done effectively in undeveloped countries. Yet another consulting job set me on the path I am traveling today.

GETTING THE FIRST CLUES

I first became involved with shark fishing when I worked as a consultant to the government of the Shah of Iran. In the mid-1970s, the shah had asked me to develop a fishery in the Persian Gulf, long before most Americans even knew where the Persian Gulf was. I suggested fishing for sharks, which were abundant in that warm-water area. Because of this consultation, I began a serious study of sharks, and the more I studied them, the more they fascinated me. Eventually, I decided to go into the shark business for myself.

Down in Panama, an area with a good shark population, I met a broker-businessman who wanted to help me market my potential products. He knew Dr. John Prudden and his work with cartilage, so he introduced me to him with the idea that Dr. Prudden might want to buy cartilage from me. Until then, I had considered cartilage just a leftover that would go into "the garbage" when I got my business underway.

When I met Dr. Prudden in 1981, he told me all about the wondrous effects of bovine cartilage. I remember saying that I just didn't believe it. Cartilage was too common to do such incredible things—stop the pain of arthritis; cure psoriasis, cancer, and inflammation; and so on. I decided to put him to the test and said, "I've got a bad back. Put me on some of your magic pills and let me see how and if these things help my back." He gave me some of his cartilage capsules, I took them, and lo and behold, the pain definitely did go away. The results were so dramatic that within three weeks, my pain had greatly diminished and my mobility had increased. Subsequently, the wife of a business associate used the same cartilage preparation to relieve an arthritic condition that prevented her from lifting her arms to shoulder height. She also smoked three packs of cigarettes a day, the smoke of which so irritated her eyes that they were constantly red and inflamed. After three weeks on the bovine cartilage preparation, the woman was able to clap her hands easily and painlessly over her head. In addition—incredibly—her inflamed eyes had turned white again.

I decided that the cartilage from my shark business would no longer be consigned to the garbage. But much remained to be done: testing, raising money, learning manufacturing techniques, and, most of all, convincing skeptics—including myself.

One day several months after my meeting with Dr. Prudden, I received a phone call from a friend of mine. "Turn on your TV!" he shouted. "Turn on the TV! On CNN every half hour they're announcing, 'Shark cartilage cures cancer.'"

I put on CNN and, sure enough, there was a news bulletin that referred to the work of a researcher at MIT. I picked up the phone, called CNN, and soon received a copy of the Associated Press release on which the bulletin was based. This in turn gave me the name of the scientist—Dr. Robert Langer. The following Monday, I called Dr. Langer and got myself invited to come up and visit.

During my visit, I said, "I don't want to be involved with any drugs since I don't have the money or resources to get FDA approval. Will I get the same results you do if I handle cartilage in its natural state very gently, using state-of-the-art processing so as not to destroy its activity, and then administer it orally?"

As I recall as clear as day, Dr. Langer told me frankly that I'd have something probably even *better* than what he had reported on because cartilage has several active components and he was measuring the antiangiogenic effect of only one protein. And prophetically, he was right; I did have something better. In 1990, Japanese researchers would prove that there are at least two proteins other than the one with which Langer was working that are also very active antiangiogenically. When using whole cartilage, we take advantage of all three, along with the immune-stimulating and anti-inflammatory capabilities of the mucopolysaccharides. When the components work in unison, there is probably a synergistic effect, which means that the result is superior to what is achieved when using each component separately. This is a major advantage of using a natural product.

GETTING DOWN TO WORK

After meeting with Dr. Langer, I headed back to Panama, where I got 200 pounds of good clean cartilage, had it frozen, and brought it back to the States. I found someone to freeze-dry the cartilage for me, then I got someone to pulverize it under nitrogen. I was handling the cartilage very gently indeed.

In 1985, I took this whole-shark-cartilage product to John Prudden and asked him to compare it to his product. Prudden sent it to the University of Arizona, where Dr. Durie (see page 49) conducted a study comparing the shark cartilage with the bovine cartilage. Dr. Durie wrote to inform me that the results with the shark-cartilage product were as good as if not slightly better than his average results with the bovine-cartilage preparation. This was later confirmed by an international pharmaceutical company's investigation, which concluded that the commercial preparation of shark cartilage is materially better as an angiogenesis inhibitor than Catrix, Prudden's bovine-cartilage preparation, and at least equal to heparin-cortisone, considered—then and now—by the traditional health-care community to be the standard for evaluating angiogenesis inhibition (see page 58).

When Dr. Durie's finding that shark cartilage is better than bovine cartilage was added to the results of the MIT study showing that shark cartilage inhibits angiogenesis and stops tumor growth and to the Folkman theory that stopping angiogenesis could halt tumor growth, the pieces began to fall into place. I had quite a convincing package by the time I was introduced to the late George Escher, M.D., of Einstein Medical College, an old-time oncologist who had also helped government research agencies set up various overseas operations for cancer research. Dr. Escher listened to me very carefully, then said, "You know, you don't have very much, but everything you've got is from a top researcher, so it certainly is worth listening to." He was so sure the work had merit that he asked my permission to send to Europe the research publications I had brought with me. He felt that my best shot at moving forward with my research was in Europe, which was a little more open than the United States to accepting a natural product as a cancer therapy.

GOING TO EUROPE

Within weeks of our discussion, Dr. Escher contacted researchers at the Institut Jules Bordet in Brussels and arranged a meeting for me with the institute's director of research. Days later, I was airborne, heading to Brussels to meet Dr. Henri Tagnon.

When I left my hotel the morning of the meeting, I really did not know what I was getting into. I had a taxi take me to the address I had been given. When we drove up, I was awed. My destination was a gigantic hospital—close to four square blocks in size. When I walked into the Hospital Bordet—of which the institute is a major part—I saw a plaque explaining that the entire facility is dedicated to the man I was about to meet.

When I met Dr. Tagnon, I was also introduced to Dr. Ghanem Atassi, his chief researcher; Dr. Serge Orloff, secretary of the International Association of Rheumatologists in Europe; two or three other associates at the lab; and a representative from the National Institutes of Health (NIH), who was visiting from Washington, D.C. They all listened to the facts I gave them—data from MIT, data proving Folkman's theory, data from Dr. Durie, and, of course, data from John Prudden. I remember very distinctly that after I had completed my presentation, Dr. Tagnon—with a big smile—said, "This is too good to believe." I fully expected him to show me the door. "But," he went on, "it's too good not to believe, and we're ready to work with you." He said he wanted to begin the research by doing a toxicity study. I pointed out that I had no money to support such work, and he said, "Don't worry about it. If it's this good, we've got the money."

And that was my first big breakthrough.

The process of turning my dream of a cure for cancer into reality began with feeding rats as much of the shark-cartilage material as they could hold. Since the rats survived these hefty daily doses for thirty days, the material was deemed to be nontoxic.

After the toxicity study, Dr. Atassi conducted experiments in which leukemia cells were injected into the peritoneal cavity (interior of the abdomen) of test animals. Three groups of test animals received oral doses of 50 to 300 milligrams of shark cartilage. Depending on the dosage they received, the test animals lived an average of 34 percent (18.4 percent to 49.4 percent) longer than did the control animals, which had been given the leukemia cells but not the shark cartilage.

Dr. Atassi next conducted studies from 1988 through 1989 that led to a practical breakthrough in the potential use of shark cartilage both as a cancer therapy and a cancer preventive. In these subsequent studies, forty mice received xenografts of a human melanoma, basically creating an induced melanoma metastasis. (A xenograft is a graft of tissue from another species.) The control animals again received no medication; the test animals received daily doses of whole dry shark cartilage administered orally as a water suspension at a rate of 1,200 milligrams per 1 kilogram of body weight. The tumor volume in both groups was periodically recorded through day twenty-eight. These measurements showed that the tumors in the untreated control animals doubled in size in twenty-one days, while the tumors in the animals that had received the shark cartilage decreased 17 percent, going from 36 milligrams on day one to 30 milligrams on day twenty-one. The Bordet researchers were astounded, claiming that these results were even more dramatic than results obtained with the most drastic chemotherapy products. And, unlike chemotherapy, shark cartilage is completely nontoxic and has no adverse side effects.

The researchers also noted with interest that almost all of the tumor growth in the untreated control animals occurred more than two weeks after the implantation. The time lag indicated that during the initial two-week period, the tumor mass was establishing the blood network needed for growth. This further confirmed that a tumor mass releases a substance that activates angiogenesis. The results so astounded the Bordet researchers that they repeated the study with slight modifications. In the second study, they waited two days after introducing the tumor mass before administering the shark cartilage in a water suspension. A time lag between the signal for the formation of the blood network and the beginning of the network's development should mean that the forty-eight-hour delay in administering the cartilage would not interfere with the expected response to the therapy.

As in the first study, the results revealed that orally administered shark cartilage stopped the growth of the tumors. In fact, tumor mass *decreased* by 40 percent, going from 41 milligrams on day one to 27 milligrams on day twenty-one. In the untreated animals, the tumor mass increased to two and a half times the original size. (The volume was 1.942 in the untreated mice and only 0.593 in those treated with dry shark cartilage.)

In both of the studies, tumor growth in the untreated control animals was roughly level until day fourteen (two weeks after tumor implantation). From approximately day fourteen through day twenty-one, a period of only one week, tumor weight increased sharply, doubling or tripling in size once the blood network was in place. The dramatic tumor growth evidenced during the third week after implantation had previously been demonstrated by Drs. Langer and Lee in their research on tumor development in the eye of a rabbit (see page 44). These results dramatically illustrated how very fast a tumor mass will grow once its blood network is in place. Logically, if the blood network can be kept from forming, cancer growth can be prevented, which suggests that shark cartilage can be used not only as a therapy but also as a preventative, or prophylactic, measure. The substantial benefits of shark cartilage truly were piling up, and other studies were showing that cancer was not the only "mystery" that shark cartilage could "solve."

THE BREAKTHROUGH EXTENDS TO ARTHRITIS

Once the initial toxicity study at Institut Jules Bordet was complete, Dr. Serge Orloff, the arthritis specialist I had met during my first meeting with Dr. Tagnon, went right to work, conducting arthritis studies with human patients (see page 117). This really shocked me because in the United States, researchers are expected to conduct a minimum of one to two years of animal studies before they can even look at a human subject. Dr. Orloff felt, however, that with a natural nontoxic material, there is no risk, just great opportunity.

While Dr. Orloff was pursuing his research, I was "networking," meeting and speaking with people, even wining and dining them, in an effort to gain support and funds. But every month or so, I would return to Brussels to see what was happening and to brainstorm about the future with the talented men at the institute.

On one of these trips to Belgium, I learned that Dr. Orloff's work had indicated that orally administered shark cartilage could control the pain associated with osteoarthritis. In the hopes of confirming this additional benefit, I logged more airtime and approached José A. Orcasita, M.D., then assistant clinical professor of internal medicine at the University of Miami School of Medicine, with a proposal for studies to confirm Orloff's results. Dr. Orcasita agreed to test shark cartilage, and the three heavily arthritic patients who completed the course of treatment responded quite favorably (see page 113). A fourth patient completed only seven-eighths of the course but also responded well. When I reported these results during my networking sessions, doubting Thomases claimed that it was all a placebo effect. To refute the possibility that the pain relief was all in the patients' minds, we undertook dog studies in Belgium with Jacques Rauis, D.V.M., in which we also attained very dramatic results (see page 120). However, despite all of these incredible results, there were many times when I felt nothing but frustration.

FIGHTING THE ESTABLISHMENT

Each day, I was uncovering more and more of the trail that had gone before me. More and more of the research that had already been conducted into angiogenesis and into cartilage's effect on tumor growth—research begun in the early 1970s—was being revealed to me. Yet, as you read this book, you are probably saying, "Why haven't I heard about it before?"

Shark cartilage is not synthesized by chemists or prescribed by physicians, so who is going to tell you about it? Certainly not the pharmaceutical companies or chemical manufacturers, who could not patent it as a drug; nor the physicians or hospitals, with their vested interests in the economics of standard medical care. Yet the information can readily be found in some of the leading *scientific* publications. Why are the scientists keeping it to themselves?

You haven't heard about shark cartilage's effect on tumor growth because cartilage is a simple, naturally occurring substance that is classified as a food supplement, not as a drug. According to the FDA, a food supplement is something that is added to a food or diet. Best known among supplements are vitamins, minerals, fiber, garlic, and unsaturated fish oils. These and all other food supplements are not considered medicinal, may make no medical claims, and are controlled by the FDA's food regulations, not by regulations for drugs.

Like any food, a food supplement must meet the FDA's cleanliness, safety, and labeling guidelines. Many of the food supplements available in stores are valuable for maintaining health and resisting disease. They are, therefore, close to medicinal in nature. However, the labels, advertising, and promotional materials may make no direct or implied claims regarding any medicinal activities; only substances classified by the FDA as "drugs" may make such claims. (See "What the FDA Does" on page 73.)

The fact that the FDA prohibits food supplements from making therapeutic or prophylactic claims does not mean food supplements are ineffective or unsafe. It may only mean that a company could not afford the $231 million or up to twenty years of effort required to get FDA approval. It definitely means that the naturally occurring supplement is not standardized; there are minor variations among batches, the same kinds of variations found in any natural organic product, such as apples or bananas. Perhaps the FDA places too much emphasis on standardization at the expense of those who might benefit from a truly effective natural product. A lack of FDA labeling sometimes leads people to believe that food supplements are merely quackery or snake-oil treatments, which is far from the truth.

Because it is apparently impossible to get FDA approval for a pure shark-cartilage product, researchers have spent the last twenty years trying to isolate, purify, and then synthesize the protein (or proteins) in shark cartilage that is responsible for the antiangiogenic activity—and have done so with limited success. It also means that I have continually been thwarted in my efforts to get the major government research organizations—the National Institutes of Health and the National Cancer Institute—involved in shark-cartilage research. The people I contacted there said that if it couldn't be done in a drug form, they weren't interested; they didn't work with natural products. The scientists whom I contacted usually would not speak on my behalf. With the peer system that exists in science,

What the FDA Does

Some Americans believe that today's government agencies resemble George Orwell's "Big Brother," watching our every move and controlling our actions. But there is at least one government agency that is more like a watchdog that barks out loud to warn the populace of danger.

The Food and Drug Administration promulgates regulations but cannot ban or recall products. What is sometimes called an FDA ban is really a court-ordered ban requested by the FDA. Only the courts can ban or recall products. What the FDA can do is seek publicity about a recall, barking loudly and clearly when it believes the public needs to be made aware of a serious risk. When the recall is completed, the FDA can ensure that the product is destroyed or suitably reconditioned and can investigate why the product was defective.

The FDA's regulations can best be summarized as follows:

- *Foods must be pure and wholesome, safe to eat, and produced under sanitary conditions.*

- *Drugs and therapeutic devices must be safe and effective when used according to their directions.*

- *Cosmetics must be safe and made from appropriate ingredients.*

- *Labeling must be truthful and informative.*

- *Drug labeling must include warnings needed for safe use.*

- *Drugs not safe for self-treatment must be restricted to sale by prescription.*

- *Drug manufacturing plants must be inspected by the FDA at least once every two years.*

- *Antibiotic drugs, insulin drugs, and coloring agents used in foods, drugs, and cosmetics must be tested in the FDA laboratories before they can be sold.*

- *Chemicals added to foods must be proven safe before they may be used.*

- *Pesticide residues that may remain on raw food crops must not exceed the safe limits set by the FDA.*

All of the FDA's regulations are concerned with either foods or drugs. The FDA defines drugs as articles "intended for use in the diagnosis, cure, mitigation, treatment or prevention of disease in man or other animals, and articles (other than food) intended to affect the structure or any function of the body of man or other animals."

With foods, the FDA is also concerned about honesty. A food is considered to be misbranded if it is purported to be for a special dietary use (if it is supposed to fulfill a dietary need that exists because of a condition such as a disease) but the label does not support the claim. The label must have specific information concerning such vitamin, mineral, and other dietary properties as the FDA secretary "determines and prescribes to be necessary in order to fully inform purchasers as to the food's value for such uses."

The FDA is truly a watchdog, striving to protect consumers from fraud and unsafe products. The effectiveness of the FDA, like the effectiveness of any watchdog, depends on people's paying attention.

scientists are afraid of making even one false step because their peers may criticize them. I, on the other hand, was raised to believe that unless you stick your neck out, you don't go forward.

Langer and Folkman, I believe, had convinced themselves that giving cartilage orally would not work because the acidic stomach would denature the angiogenesis-inhibiting protein, which would, therefore, be of no effect. They probably never even tried it. I pushed ahead. My researchers administered shark cartilage orally and—lo and behold—there was a positive effect. It did work, first on mice and eventually on people.

PREPARING SHARK CARTILAGE FOR ITS NEW ROLE

The oral (and later rectal) administration of shark cartilage depended on creating a product that was as pure as possible. (See "Components of Dried Shark Cartilage" on page 76.) Because of this, I handled much of the planning, research, testing, and management involved in the development of a viable shark-cartilage product for humans. Finding a way to dry and then pulverize cartilage without rendering the protein fibers ineffective was one of the major problems. The normal drying, pulverization, and sterilization processes with their excessive heat as well as the treatments that utilize solvents or chemicals often denature the active protein in cartilage and render the protein and therefore the cartilage therapeutically valueless. Proteins are easily denatured by heat and other manufacturing processes and by various chemicals like solvents and acids that are designed to remove fats and other unneeded components.

The central strands of protein that make up the heart of shark cartilage are among the largest proteins produced by any cells. It is these strands, called macroproteins, that appear to carry the angiogenesis inhibitor; and it is these strands, so prevalent in shark cartilage, that give the cartilage 1,000 times the antiangiogenesis effect of mammalian cartilage. When looking at a piece of shark cartilage, you can see the strands containing the antiangiogenesis inhibitor in the matrices of all the components. (See Figure 1.3 on page 32.)

Components of Dried Shark Cartilage

Simple chemical analysis shows that unadulterated dry shark cartilage is approximately 41 percent ash, 39 percent protein, 12 percent carbohydrates, 7 percent water, less than 1 percent fiber, and less than 0.3 percent fat. The ash is 60 percent calcium and phosphorus at a ratio of two parts calcium to one part phosphorus. Almost no heavy metals are found in the ash because without blood vessels in the cartilage, there is no way for the heavy metals often found in minimal amounts in shark meat to be deposited in the shark cartilage. The high levels of calcium and phosphorus are the result of calcification of the cartilage, especially of the backbone cartilage.

Although the protein that is the angiogenesis inhibitor is diluted to some degree by the calcium, phosphorus, carbohydrates, and other natural components, the diluents play an active role in disease control. The mucopolysaccharides in the carbohydrates stimulate the immune system, which works synergistically with the protein in fighting disease, and the organic calcium and phosphorus are used metabolically as nutrients.

These strands are very tough and almost impossible to pulverize, yet they are the material essential to antiangiogenesis. It required extensive research and development to learn how to pulverize these strands without denaturing the protein from which they are made. In addition, the abundant water content of cartilage (cartilage is more than 85 percent water) and the way in which the water is bound within the cartilage also make drying difficult and costly. Heat must be used sparingly since excessive heat is damaging.

In shark cartilage, at least one of the proteins active as an angiogenesis inhibitor is denatured if processing temperatures are elevated. Furthermore, both the cartilage and the protein within it are inactivated if they are treated with solvents like acetone or submitted to strong acids for extended periods. Fortunately, there is practically no fat attached to shark cartilage, so solvent extraction as a processing step is unnecessary. In the processing of bovine cartilage, which normally has a fairly high amount of fat clinging to it, solvent extraction is needed to keep the product from turning rancid. The acetone used to remove the fat connected to bovine cartilage denatures the already modest amount of angiogenesis-inhibiting protein.

Particle size, which is dependent on how well pulverized a material is, is another consideration. Shark cartilage must be absorbed into the system as quickly as possible to prevent the protein from being digested by proteolytic enzymes. If digested by these enzymes, the protein is broken down into its constituent amino acids, which are not effective in antiangiogenesis. The preformed protein, rather, is what is effective as the angiogenesis inhibitor. Shark-cartilage powder must therefore be finely enough pulverized to be quickly absorbed into the body system as a suspension of preformed protein. Experience has shown that at least 90 percent must pass through a 200-mesh screen for maximum effectiveness. This is finer than most talcum powders.

I spent many years, much effort, and a great deal of money getting the cartilage ready for use. The powdered cartilage I finally gave researchers was the best possible material with which they could conduct their studies. Many other major medical breakthroughs have resulted from the same process— an independent researcher working without public research funds out of a dedication to accomplish something in which he or she truly believed.

My dedication to accomplish what I believe in has kept me going.

After years of knocking on doors, networking, and nagging, shark-cartilage proponents finally attracted the interest of several traditional researchers and medical practitioners. It was the work of these people that allowed things to come together just as 1992 was beginning.

First, on Christmas Eve 1991, I received a "use patent," which indicates not only that we did it first but that the process really works. (See "The Best Christmas Present" on page 79.) You can get a patent only if you can show concrete results. You can't do it on hot air; it has to be based on hard evidence, on facts.

Next, shortly after receiving the patent, I was able to interest Roger Jacobs, Ph.D., director of the Surgical Research Laboratory at Metropolitan Hospital Center in New York City, in experimentally evaluating shark cartilage for antitumor characteristics. Dr. Jacobs conducted a pilot experiment in which rats with developing liver-tumor implants received suspensions of milled shark cartilage by intraperitoneal injection. In both gross and histologic tissue examination, it was found that the tumor growth appeared to be unaffected by the presence of the cartilage. In addition, fluid had accumulated in the peritoneal cavity and body fat appeared to have been lost, effects that were not observed in the untreated tumor-bearing controls.

In this small-animal experiment, rapidly growing tumors were used. However, when the tumor is well-established with a developed capillary blood supply, the antiangiogenic properties of shark cartilage might not be adequate to significantly slow tumor development over a short period of time. The presence of shark cartilage prior to and during the development of a tumor might inhibit angiogenesis before it has a chance to start and may thus prevent tumor development. Dr. Jacobs is

The Best
Christmas Present

It is estimated that only about three patents have ever been issued to the health-food industry. Patents are difficult to obtain for health foods because hard evidence about such foods' effectiveness is often not available. Representatives of the health-food industry also do not usually seek patents, as do representatives of the pharmaceutical industry. Many food supplements are effective products, but proving their effectiveness is difficult, and sometimes test procedures don't exist.

Since the evidence of shark cartilage's ability to inhibit angiogenesis can be proven by the CAM assay and the results of the xenograft studies conducted at the Institut Jules Bordet, I did apply for a patent. The patent was issued to me on Christmas Eve 1991. It reads in part: "This invention relates generally to a method of, and a dosage unit for, inhibiting angiogenesis or vascularization in an animal having an intestinal wall utilizing an effective amount of shark cartilage, particularly finely divided shark cartilage, for passing through the intestinal wall as a suspension for inhibiting interalia, tumor growth and metastasis, in particular Kaposi sarcoma; arthritis, in particular rheumatoid arthritis; diabetic retinopathy and neovascular glaucoma; psoriasis and inflammatory diseases with vascular component."

This patent will give the consumer protection against the "copycat" products that often haunt successful health-food products not protected by patent. Copycat products—the manufacturers of which are spurred by the desire to make a profit—may not be produced with the care needed to assure quality. The products may not even undergo the testing necessary to assure effectiveness. This is a particulary serious problem with a shark-cartilage product since the cartilage requires proper processing to ensure quality and reliability. The proper method of processing shark cartilage took months—if not years—to perfect. As the patent says, "It will be understood that the shark cartilage useful in the method of the present invention may be prepared by any suitable means or process to result in shark cartilage that is substantially pure shark cartilage, substantially free from adhering tissue."

With the patent issued on Christmas Eve, I received the best Christmas present I could have, but the United States Patent Office also gave a gift to all hopeful and potential users of shark cartilage. The patent will legally stop copycat manufacturers and distributors so that maximum effort can be devoted to improving the quality of shark cartilage to provide its users with maximum benefit.

therefore now conducting preliminary "preload" experiments in which shark cartilage is being administered intraperitoneally to rats two days prior to the implanting of the tumors. A preload experiment has the added advantage of giving the cartilage more time in which to work. I believe that this is important because a biological product such as shark cartilage doesn't work as quickly as a concentrated chemical works. In addition to the different experimental procedure, the cartilage Dr. Jacobs is now using has been processed differently.

Dr. Jacobs told me that in one of five animals bearing tumors and also given cartilage, the tumor was clearly smaller than those in the untreated controls. In three, the tumors may have been smaller but the interpretation was difficult. In all the animals given shark cartilage, there was an inflammatory response similar to that in the first experiment.

Dr. Jacobs says, "These experiments are very preliminary, and without additional experiments, including repeats of the previous studies, no conclusion can be reached. Additional experimentation is necessary to clarify these results and to establish if in fact shark cartilage has antitumor properties. It is only through additional experimentation that we can determine whether shark cartilage can be used in the treatment of human cancers."

The year 1991 was also the year the National Cancer Institute's people finally agreed to meet with me. The National Cancer Institute (NCI) is one of the National Institutes of Health (NIH), a federal agency that conducts and supports biomedical research into the causes, cure, and prevention of diseases. NIH conducts research in its own laboratories and awards grants and contracts to universities and other private research facilities. In fact, a large number of so-called independent investigators are funded by NIH grants. Separate institutes are concerned with various conditions such as cancer; heart, lung, and blood diseases; aging; and mental health. NCI, the largest of the institutes, was established by an act of Congress in 1937 and is the federal government's official agency for research into cancer and its treatment. A great deal of this research is conducted in the Laboratory of Tumor Cell Biology, where Robert Gallo, M.D., is chief.

I met with Dr. Gallo and approximately thirty of his colleagues in what promised to be a truly major step forward. These professionals—the cream of the crop—listened to me. Oh, there were critics among them, but Gallo put them in their place, and at the end of my presentation, I received a standing ovation from this orthodox medical group.

Although these NCI representatives promised to begin studies utilizing shark cartilage in the treatment of Kaposi's sarcoma (see "Kaposi's Sarcoma" on page 82) and agreed to work in coordination with me, sharing any results, they reneged on the promise less than three months later. And I

Kaposi's Sarcoma

In the 1980s, when the AIDS (acquired immune deficiency syndrome) epidemic was first being publicized, the name "Kaposi's sarcoma" burst upon the consciousness of scores of Americans, many of whom thought it was a newly discovered or at least newly named disease. Nothing could have been further from the truth.

Kaposi's sarcoma (KS) is actually a form of cancer that was first identified in 1872 by Moritz Kaposi. In KS, odd-shaped tumor cells cling to the linings of small blood vessels. Unchecked, the growths will eventually clog the vessels. Affected limbs may become swollen, and affected organs may become congested and enlarged.

KS is relatively common in Africa, where AIDS is believed to have originated. One researcher has postulated that hygienic practices explain the high incidence of the disease there. In some parts of equatorial Africa, about 10 percent of all cancers are KS. In that part of the world, the disease often strikes children, for whom it is particularly deadly as it is often accompanied by enormously swollen lymph nodes in the neck.

In the United States prior to 1980, the disease was so rare that only one in one million people was afflicted with it. Those afflicted were elderly men of Ashkenazi (Eastern European) Jewish or Mediterranean Italian background. It rarely touched women or young men. New York University's Cancer Registry recorded no cases of KS in patients under fifty at Bellevue Hospital from 1970 through 1979. In the men that were afflicted, the course of the disease was usually slow and the characteristic brown or purple spots were confined to the legs. KS was usually treated successfully, and there were few fatalities.

Kaposi's sarcoma became slightly more commonplace after the first successful kidney transplant in 1950. Organ recipients receive immune-suppressant drugs to prevent the body from rejecting the transplanted organ, leaving the recipients susceptible to KS. It was, therefore, apparent that Kaposi's sarcoma is an immune-suppression disease, or "opportunistic cancer," a cancer that develops because of the host's lack of normal defenses. When treatment with the immune-suppressant drugs was discontinued, the KS disappeared. However, an ever-increasing incidence of the disease would soon be apparent.

In 1981, the Communicable Disease Center in Atlanta, Georgia, first began to receive reports of KS in young men who had engaged in homosexual activities. This was the harbinger of what was to become the AIDS epidemic. Approximately 25 percent of AIDS patients are diagnosed with KS. However, autopsies reveal KS lesions in 90 percent of those who die of AIDS. The condition is more common among male homosexuals with AIDS than among other people with AIDS.

Neither AIDS nor Kaposi's sarcoma responds to conventional treatment. Kaposi's will respond temporarily to a variety of chemotherapeutic drugs and to interferon, an anticancer and antiviral substance. In March 1992, the journal "Science" reported that two new drugs seemed promising; both prevent angiogenesis, which is necessary to the development of KS.

The lesions of Kaposi's sarcoma are formed from endothelial cells, the cells that line blood vessels, which are the very cells kept from developing by shark cartilage and other angiogenesis inhibitors. Since KS lesions are made of endothelial cells and shark cartilage apparently inhibits the development of these cells, use of shark cartilage should show positive results for those with KS. Shark cartilage should also be effective because KS lesions are heavily vascularized and, as we have seen, shark cartilage is an effective vascularization inhibitor.

I have, in fact, recently learned about a man who is believed to be the first to have a remission of KS. Michael Callanan, author of "Surviving AIDS," was diagnosed as having

AIDS in the early 1980s. Eventually, KS lesions covered more than two-thirds of his lungs. The chemotherapy prescribed to fight his KS had such "horrible" side effects that Michael called a halt to them. Two months later, he learned of an opening in a clinical trial being conducted by Eric Fleishman, M.D., of Los Angeles. Michael entered the program and began taking shark cartilage. He also elected to undergo radiation therapy despite warnings that "it was not a very good idea" (radiation might further compromise his immune system) and that he should "not expect anything." Neither the radiologist nor the technician knew that he was taking shark cartilage.

Michael's right lung was treated in sessions using 1,000 rads, a relatively low dose. When the course of treatment was completed, that lung was completely clear, but Michael's left lung had gotten worse. The left lung was also treated with radiation for ten days, after which both lungs were completely clear of KS lesions.

Health-care professionals involved with Michael believe that the shark cartilage acted as a radiation potentiator. Further evidence of cartilage's ability to augment the effect of radiation came when Michael had treatment for lesions on his legs. The plan had been for him to receive a normal dose of 2,000 rads. At 1,200 rads, a dose normally free from side effects, he began to exhibit radiation burns. Michael, therefore, urges those taking shark cartilage to inform their radiologists. He also recommends that shark-cartilage users begin with low doses of radiation.

learned about the revised decision only as a result of a telephone conversation with an NCI employee.

A *New York Times* reporter had called to talk to me about my patent and seemed interested when I mentioned that NCI was becoming involved in the shark-cartilage studies. When I hung up the phone, I decided to let Dr. Gallo and his associates know that the *Times* reporter might want to ask them some questions. I never got that far.

My phone call was handled by an NCI representative who told me that the shark-cartilage research would not be pursued. I was told that even though NIH in general seeks cures for the diseases it researches, NCI does not deal in "cures" for cancer but only in the "mechanisms" of cancer. Furthermore, NCI people felt that it would "serve" my "self-interests" if the organization appeared to be interested in shark cartilage.

"But what if it works?" I replied. "What if shark cartilage can actually stop the growth of cancer? Isn't it worth further consideration?" The answer was that the decision not to move forward with testing at NCI had been made and was final. End of subject.

FEARS OF BLINDNESS AND IGNORANCE

If you look at the history of research into cancer therapies, you see that when people who are outside of the medical establishment try to present a more effective treatment for cancer, they are labeled "charlatans," "quacks," and worse. This is especially true when the researchers work directly with humans. Just think of Dr. Max Gerson, Dr. Stanislaw Burzynski, and Mr. Harry Hoxsey. These gentlemen provided literally hundreds of cancer-patient case studies demonstrating the effectiveness of their treatments. Instead of the accuracy of their claims being investigated, their characters were attacked and their work ignored.

Gerson, Burzynski, and Hoxsey—all three medical "outsiders"—tried to get members of the scientific community to evaluate their results; instead, their studies were labeled simply "anecdotal." Their data didn't come from controlled experiments; one person simply reported that he had seen something work with positive results. It may be "anecdotal" to read about a forty-year-old man or woman who has had his or her cancer reversed, but it's not so anecdotal if that forty-year-old person is someone you know and love.

I suspect that the system that quashed Gerson, Burzynski, and Hoxsey is perhaps still in place today. While some may call this suspicion paranoia, the historical reality is that pioneers in science face an uphill battle. I believe that getting the information in this book to the public is well worth that battle. All I ask is that the facts presented herein be the focus of attention and that I be judged on their validity.

4.

Clinical Trials

It has been estimated that only 10–20% of all procedures currently used in medical practice have been shown to be efficacious by controlled trial.

Office of Technology Assessment
Assessing the Efficacy and Safety of Medical Technologies

I 've talked—and am talking—to as many people as I can, and I have been able to network with physicians who, after reading the evidence I gave them, could see the potential of shark-cartilage therapy in an arena in which other defenders are losing the battle. Since 1989, these physicians have been working with me to bring their patients a new approach to cancer therapy.

WORK WITH HUMANS BEGINS

In Costa Rica, which has both a large shark population and a factory for the processing of shark cartilage, Carlos Luís Alpizar, M.D., is the head of the geriatrics program in the social security hospital. He was familiar with the angiogenesis theory behind the use of shark cartilage and with some of the shark-cartilage research. When called upon in the late 1980s to treat a patient with an inoperable abdominal tumor that was the size of a large grapefruit, Dr. Alpizar was quite pessimistic about the patient's chances for survival. He felt that the patient was obviously in a terminal stage of the disease. With no other avenues open to him, Dr. Alpizar asked for and was given experimental quantities of dry shark cartilage.

This dry cartilage was taken orally by the patient at the rate of 12 grams per day in three equal portions before meals. No other treatment was used since Dr. Alpizar held no hope for the survival of the patient. The tumor, measured by sonographic procedures, stopped growing within a month. After six months of constant shark-cartilage treatment, the grapefruit-sized tumor had been reduced to the size of a walnut. The patient regained his appetite, was again able to function, and was, after these six months, able to return to a normal life. My excitement was second only to that of the patient.

Armed with my enthusiasm and with these impressive results, I sought other physicians who would expand upon Dr. Alpizar's important work. In research—especially in research on advanced cancer patients—it is difficult to get patients to whom you can administer only a test product. Both doctors and patients are obviously reluctant, desiring only the best available treatment in order to afford the patient the best chance for survival. Using only test materials that have a minimal track record is really experimenting on patients. But as AIDS patients often proclaim, "Make us guinea pigs. Give us the drugs. Let us decide." I was fortunate enough to find a physician who shared the same view as that held by AIDS patients.

VISION IN MEXICO

In 1991, I was able to enlist the cooperation of the directors of the Ernesto Contreras Hospital in Tijuana, Mexico. People have mentioned to me that the Contreras Hospital is considered the "over-the-border treatment center." I know it is surrounded by controversy, but the plain fact is the physicians there are willing to work with innovative techniques that show better promise than do the conventional strategies. It's controversial, yes, but many of history's pioneering scientists have been labeled controversial—men like Galileo, Louis Pasteur, Joseph Lister, and even Jonas Salk. (See "Jonas Salk Fights More Than Polio" on page 90.)

In Mexico, Ernesto Contreras, Sr., M.D., has a reputation of being somewhat of a "saint" because of his clinical abilities and willingness to treat indigent patients without charge. A medical practitioner for more than fifty years, he has devoted the past thirty years to finding less aggressive but more effective alternatives to the conventional treatment of cancer. He and his sons—Ernesto Contreras, Jr., M.D., and Francisco Contreras, M.D., who both specialize in cancer treatment—run the fifty-bed Contreras Hospital, which has a radiology department, a clinical laboratory, and a staff with extensive experience in treating cancer patients.

The physicians at the Contreras Hospital had been using shark cartilage but in very low amounts, and frankly, they weren't getting any positive results. The three Contrerases were, however, receptive to the concept of using cartilage, so when we discussed the possibilities of using a higher dosage level and a more active product, they were willing to try. The Contrerases agreed to treat ten cancer patients free of charge. The patients would be chosen based on the doctors' estimate that these patients had little chance of surviving for six months because they were all in the late stages (Stage III or Stage IV) of the disease. Ernesto, Jr., medical director of the hospital, would provide hospital, medical, and nursing care with no fees, and I would provide an advanced form of shark-cartilage mate-

Jonas Salk Fights More Than Polio

Ask an American to name a famous scientist who is alive today and the chances are "Jonas Salk" will be the answer. Salk, developer of the polio vaccine, may be well-known now, but in 1952, he was an unknown laboratory researcher. A year later, he was mired in national controversy. Much of the controversy revolved around his use of killed polio viruses to form his injection. Not only was it considered very risky, but many scientists—chief among them Albert B. Sabin, who developed the Sabin oral polio vaccine—did not believe that use of killed viruses would provide permanent immunity to the disease.

Dr. W. Lloyd Aycock of Harvard University was one of many who warned against the polio vaccine. He felt that the need was to find and vaccinate only those children who were susceptible to the disease. "Nature does a better job of immunizing than we could hope to do artificially," he said.

Dr. Thomas Francis, Jr., who was chosen by the National Foundation for Infantile Paralysis to direct the field trials and pass judgment on the Salk polio vaccine, was acutely aware of the controversy. He said, "I dread the time when the scientist must have the concurrence of all his colleagues and competitors."

In "The Virus Hunters," a book by Greer Williams, Salk is described as the "Man in the Long White Coat" who had to work "shoulder to shoulder with the promoters and organizers . . . who want to put useful knowledge across with the utmost impact." Because of his association with such men, Salk was considered a "publicity hound," a reputation that earned him the scorn of many of his colleagues. "The New York Times" reported that one of Salk's colleagues had said to Salk: "The only time I see you these days is on television."

Salk had become involved in vaccine research in 1943, when he joined Dr. Francis in the fieldtesting of a vaccine against two strains of influenza. It was this testing that had first demonstrated the potency of a killed virus in producing antibodies. Once the potency issue was resolved, the pressing question became how to achieve the same kind of lasting immunity that was induced with the attenuated live-virus smallpox vaccine.

Salk's work on the polio vaccine was a matter of following the trail of clues and putting together the pieces. The pieces consisted of:

- *The discovery in 1951 that there are three different types of polio virus, each producing specific antibodies.*

- *The information that antibodies against polio can protect against paralysis, which was based on the discovery that the virus shows up in the bloodstream before any symptoms of paralytic polio appear, anywhere from five to thirty-one days after the injection.*

- *The production of marginally successful killed-virus vaccines by two other investigators.*

- *The discovery of a method for growing polio viruses in ordinary tissue so that they could be cultivated in sufficient quantity to produce a vaccine.*

Salk's ability to put the pieces together was often scorned. It was said that he was merely using other researchers' ideas and that he was in the right place at the right time. Salk, who did the bulk of his work when he was research professor and director of the Virus Research Laboratories at the University of Pittsburgh with a large lab and a staff of fifty, was in an excellent position to "put the ingredients together" to make a vaccine. "It is easy enough to say that if he had not created his vaccine, someone else would have done the job," wrote Robert Coughlan in the June 20, 1955, issue of "Life." Coughlan points out, however, that if people had waited for others to "prove the superiority of their method (as someday they may) it would have been at the cost of thousands who in the meantime would have been crippled or killed for lack of any protection."

To test the antibody production that would result from his vaccine, Salk decided in 1952 to try the vaccine at a home for crippled children. Because the children had already had polio, they were presumably immune. He first tested the children for existing polio antibodies so that he could make comparisons. When antibodies existed, they rose to even higher levels after vaccination.

Salk's work led him to conclude, "It is possible, with non-infectious material, to approximate, and perhaps to exceed, the level of antibody produced by infection." Many virologists questioned whether he was selling them a bill of goods.

But Salk apparently completely believed in what he was doing. He vaccinated himself, his wife, and their three sons— nine-year-old Peter, six-year-old Darrell, and three-year-old Jonathan. Each of the Salks evidenced a dramatic increase in antibody level. Then, in 1953, in an affluent suburb of Pittsburgh, 474 children were vaccinated on the assumption that where soap and water were used abundantly, natural immunity to polio would be at its lowest. Indeed, when the children were tested to determine their pre-injection antibody levels, 60 percent showed no detectable antibodies. Following vaccination, the antibody level soared.

At this time, Dr. Albert Mitzer of Michael Reese Hospital in Chicago announced that he had used Salk's method of killing the polio virus without success. Other scientists around the nation were put off by the certainty of Salk's superiors, who said that anyone who could not reproduce Salk's results had not followed his methods. Professional jealousy seemed rampant.

In addition, scientists who had been working on the Immunization Committee of the National Foundation for Infantile Paralysis felt that they were being by-passed. Others wanted more time to confirm Salk's claims in other labs; they wanted to set up a consortium of universities that would share their findings with one another. Dr. Joseph A. Bell, an epidemiologist with the Public Health Service's National Institute of Infectious and Allergic Diseases, drafted the standards that would be used for the field trials—standards in which every drop of the vaccine would be triple-tested for safety, first by the manufacturing laboratory, then by Salk's lab, and finally by the Health Service's lab. But as summer sore throats sent ripples of fear through every parent in the nation, the threat of extensive delay caused an uproar. Bell resigned during the ensuing dispute.

The field trials were bogged down in bickering until 1954. Some epidemiologists insisted on a double-blind study with a placebo; neither the doctor nor the children would know who was getting what. But denying half the children the real vaccine and its benefits presented a moral dilemma to other scientists. Still others felt that the National Foundation could not be trusted to run the tests since an organization committed to the conquest of polio might not be impartial.

Finally, by mid-May, the triple-tested vaccination had been fieldtested—642,360 first and second graders had received the first of three shots. Some received the killed virus, some received a placebo, and some received neither (they were just pricked). Polio rates in the test areas dropped to 40 percent below rates of previous years.

Further fieldtesting as well as manufacturing problems revealed that the vaccine's ability to produce antibodies was variable and that some batches were "essentially devoid of antigenic activity." According to Williams in "The Virus Hunters," "The Salk vaccine was anything but a standardized product."

As the debate raged over whether or not to let Salk continue his work, one participant said, "Those who would prevent [the vaccine's] use must be prepared to be haunted *for life by the crippled bodies of little children who would have been saved from paralysis had they been permitted to receive the Salk Vaccine."*

The Salk Vaccine was finally distributed commercially in 1955. At this time, an article in the magazine section of "The New York Times" postulated, "The real proof will be in the record." The record has, of course, spoken. The Salk Vaccine eliminated a tragic problem, and Jonas Salk became the best known of any of the scientists who had been involved in the experimentation.

rial without charge. We were hoping to get a 5-, 10-, 15-, 20-percent response. The initial plan called for four months of cartilage treatment to be administered to ten patients. Dr. Ernesto Contreras, Jr., elected to treat the chosen patients with 30 grams of the cartilage material daily in the form of a water suspension. For female patients, half the daily dose would be given via a retention enema and half would be introduced into the vaginal body cavity. Male patients would receive two retention enemas. These methods of treatment would allow the protein of the shark cartilage to be quickly absorbed into the system.

It is essential that the protein content of the cartilage be absorbed before it is digested by enzymes. Once digested, the protein is broken down into its constituent amino acids, which are not effective as angiogenesis inhibitors. Absorption can be accomplished from the intestine via oral administration or from any other body cavity or part.

Therapeutic agents are administered in any of several ways in order to achieve rapid absorption. These agents are typically administered orally, as are pills, or rectally, as are antiseasickness suppositories. They may also be administered via skin patches that allow the agent to be absorbed directly into the skin. All of these methods require that the particle size of the therapeutic agent be small enough to pass through a membrane. The active protein in shark cartilage is small enough to be administered in any of these ways.

Dr. Ernesto Contreras, Jr., had observed that when treating advanced cancer patients, enzymes and other nutrients are often more effective when given via retention enemas than when administered orally. He therefore decided to treat the ten patients by introducing the shark cartilage into the body cavities from which the cartilage would be absorbed into the blood system as directly and quickly as possible. According to scientists at the National Cancer Institute, patients with advanced cancer may experience changes in the functional capability of the digestive tract. In these cases, the normally acidic stomach frequently becomes abnormally alkaline with an accompanying reduction in absorptive capability. Dr. Contreras's choice of rectal administration would circumvent this problem. In addition, this method of introduction has the advantage of utilizing large blood vessels (often seen as hemorrhoids) designed to conserve body fluids, specifically the fluids used in the process of digestion. These blood vessels, which act like highly efficient sponges in absorbing excess water, provide a very efficient route for the administration of shark-cartilage suspensions. The vaginal cavity is just a convenient second cavity that Dr. Contreras decided to use.

Eventually, eight patients were involved in the Contreras study; of the original ten, one dropped out of the study and one died early on. The eight remaining advanced cancer patients were looked upon as terminal, yet over a two-month period, a positive response would be seen in seven of them. In the seven cases, there would be a reduction in tumor size of 30 to 100 percent. And these results with the terminal cancer patients would be directly due to the shark-cartilage therapy and only the shark-cartilage therapy.

Case Histories

Each of the eight patients was first evaluated by Ernesto Contreras, Jr., and taught how to self-administer the cartilage. The patients were then given packets containing premeasured 15-gram doses of a highly concentrated experimental shark cartilage to be mixed just prior to administration with two-thirds cup of water at body temperature. A total of two packets (30 grams) was administered daily using a soft-sided plastic syringe-like device with a two-inch-long enema head. The patients were seen every week by a nurse and were given additional packets of cartilage material. Every second week, Dr. Contreras, Jr., evaluated the patients' progress and met with the patients if necessary.

The eight cases consisted of:

- A forty-eight-year-old woman with a Stage III inoperable locally advanced uterine cervix cancer with invasion to the bladder. Earlier doses of radiation had not helped; the woman had ulcerations and considerable pain related to the tumor. Following seven weeks of shark-cartilage therapy, the pain was largely gone and the tumor was 80 percent smaller. After eleven weeks of treatment, there was a complete (100-percent) reduction in tumor size; all that remained was scar tissue, which could be palpated (examined by touching). The pain was completely gone.

- A fifty-year-old woman with a vaginal hemangioma the size of a large grapefruit, five inches by five inches, that was persistent even after a hysterectomy. A partial vaginectomy and maximum doses of external and internal radiation had not helped. After seven weeks of shark-cartilage treatment, the tumor was at least 60 percent smaller and no bleeding was evident. After eleven weeks, the tumor was down to the size of a small orange. This case is considered one of the most significant in the study because it is a clear-cut example of antiangiogenesis. A hemangioma is a continually growing blood pocket or vessel. Though not a malignant tumor, a hemangioma may be life-threatening because if it opens, the victim can bleed to death. It is also quite similar to a Kaposi's sarcoma lesion, giving us hope that shark cartilage will work well with that condition.

- A thirty-two-year-old woman with a Stage IV (very advanced) uterine cervix cancer with kidney blockage, which necessitated the constant use of a catheter in the urethra. Treatment with shark cartilage was started as a last resort; in cases such as this, death is considered practically a certainty. After seven weeks, the tumor was at least 40 percent smaller, the urethral catheter was no longer needed, the pain was almost gone, and the patient was eating better and starting to gain weight. At eleven weeks, the tumor was 60 percent smaller.

- A forty-eight-year-old man, the only male patient in the study, with a Stage III very large inoperable soft-tissue sarcoma covering the entire back of his right thigh. There had been partial response to radiation therapy, but the tumor had continued to grow rapidly. After seven weeks of cartilage therapy, there was no externally visible relief. After nine weeks, Ernesto Contreras, Jr., reluctantly decided that surgical removal of the tumor was necessary. During the operation, Francisco Contreras, the surgeon, found that the entire center of the tumor—more than 60 percent of the mass—had gelatinized and necrosed. The tumor was breaking down from the inside out and there was no metastasis to the lung, as is so often the case with this type of cancer.

- A thirty-eight-year-old female with a residual tumor after a total hysterectomy for uterine cervix cancer. The tumor had not responded to maximum doses of both internal and external radiation. The patient was in generally poor physical condition and was experiencing many symptoms, including significant pain related to her cancer. After six weeks on shark-cartilage therapy, subjective improvement was clearly evidenced. The pain was largely gone as were the majority of other symptoms, and the woman elected to stop treatment at seven weeks. However, at eleven weeks, tumors were discovered in both of the woman's lungs. This indicates that cartilage therapy probably has to be continued at least until all tumor signs are gone.

- A sixty-two-year-old female with bone metastasis to the right sacroiliac region from a previously treated uterine cervix cancer. The metastasis developed in an area that had been radiated. Following nine weeks of shark-cartilage therapy, the tumor was at least 80 percent smaller. At eleven weeks, all signs of the tumor were gone, and the patient was considered cured.

- A thirty-six-year-old female with a Stage IV peritoneal carcinoma from a colon primary cancer. Exploratory surgery had confirmed the diagnosis of inoperable cancer, and the patient had been given little chance of survival. Following seven weeks of shark-cartilage treatment, the patient developed an abdominal-wall abscess that required a second surgical procedure. During the surgery, the tumor was found to be 80 percent smaller, and most of the remaining tumor was found to be gelatinized. This was, of course, due to tumor necrosis, indicating another successfully treated case. At eleven weeks, the patient was tumor-free and was considered by the doctors to be a "miracle cure."

- A forty-five-year-old female with a bilateral inflammatory breast cancer with skin and chest-wall invasion. This was the only patient who did not respond to the cartilage. After six weeks, the lack of response was evident, and the therapy was terminated.

How, you ask, could the seven tumors have been caused to necrose? It is simple enough to understand that an angiogenesis inhibitor can effectively stop *further* growth of a tumor mass, but how can an existing tumor mass be *shrunk* by an angiogenesis inhibitor?

The answer lies in the fact that the blood network of a tumor is fragile, decidedly more fragile than a normal blood network. Since the vessels in a tumor network are constantly breaking down, they always have to be replaced. If an inhibitor of angiogenesis like shark cartilage—or, more precisely, like the protein that naturally occurs in shark cartilage—can stop the formation of replacement vessels, rapid necrosis can and will occur, as seen in these case studies.

The Contreras's study of the eight patients has largely been concluded. The responses detailed above are quite startling; seven cancer patients who previously had little or no hope of survival now bless the Contreras doctors and shark cartilage.

Further Mexican Studies

In Mexico, results were released in May 1992 from preliminary clinical studies conducted by Roscoe L. Van Zandt, M.D. Dr. Van Zandt, a gynecologist in Arlington, Texas, who works part-time at the Hoxsey Clinic in Tijuana, Mexico, reported that eight women with advanced breast tumors had received 30 to 60 grams of orally administered shark cartilage daily. In all eight patients, after six to eight weeks, the tumors had significantly reduced in size. Upon examination of some of the tumors, it was obvious that the internal tissue had changed color from pink to gray, a sign of necrosis. In three cases, the tumors had become encapsulated, and in two cases in which the tumors had become attached to the chest wall, they had become detached and free-floating. According to Dr. Van Zandt, attached tumors rarely if ever become detached since once they are attached, they erode the bone of the chest wall. In addition to these eight breast-cancer cases, two women with uterine fibroid tumors had experienced a disappearance of their tumors. None of these ten cases is definitive and the results from all are preliminary, but the cases do show exciting possibilities and the need for additional studies.

THE PANAMA PROJECT

A team of health-care professionals in Panama led by Ella Ferguson, Ph.D., has also been investigating shark cartilage's effect on cancer. In one case, a forty-three-year-old male with terminal pulmonary cancer and metastases to the bone and brain received shark-cartilage capsules beginning in November 1991. No other therapy was used because it was believed that conventional medicine would not be effective.

During the period between November 1991 and January 1992, there was noticeable improvement in ventilatory capacity (respiration). The patient stopped feeling pain in his chest and in his left and right hips. However, cerebral metastasis continued, and the shark-cartilage dosage was increased to 30 grams daily, rectally administered.

In the middle of February 1992, the patient began complaining of bad headaches and double vision. The dosage was again increased, this time to 60 grams daily. Following seventy-two hours of increased dosage, the pain diminished, the double vision cleared, and the symptoms did not recur. The disappearance of these symptoms indicates that the cerebral tumor may have been shrinking.

In another case, a patient with an advanced liver tumor received 60 grams of shark cartilage daily in the form of four 15-gram retention enemas. Over an eight-week period with no treatment other than the shark cartilage, the patient experienced complete remission of the tumor. I had personally seen this patient before treatment began and held little hope. When I saw him after eight weeks of treatment, he was gaining weight and looking quite robust.

WORK IN CUBA DRAWS MEDIA ATTENTION

One of the most exciting of our clinical trials was recently conducted in Cuba. This study not only proved to be a gold mine of information, but it was featured on CBS-TV's *60 Minutes* early in 1993, thus giving my work tremendous visibility.

The *60 Minutes* investigative reporters had been conducting a diligent study of the uses of shark cartilage for almost a year. In January 1993, cameramen and reporters accompanied me to Cuba, where they witnessed the dramatic results of a trial involving twenty-seven terminal cancer patients.

I had first made the Cuban connection in 1992, when representatives of the Cuban government invited me to conduct a study with civilian patients in one of Cuba's modern and fully equipped military hospitals. Twenty-seven terminal cancer patients, all classified as either Stage III or Stage IV, were chosen to participate. Most had previously undergone surgery, radiation, chemotherapy, or a combination of treatments without success. The patients were admitted to a fully staffed clinic adjacent to the hospital for the duration of the study, thereby ensuring standardization of the protocol and allowing for extensive laboratory testing (ultrasound, CAT scans, X-rays, blood work-ups) and record-keeping. When clinical trials are conducted outside of a hospital, as they often are in the United States, it is very difficult to ensure that patients follow the correct procedures.

According to the procedure in the Cuban study, each patient received 60 grams a day of a 100-percent-pure shark-cartilage product processed according to the patent discussed on pages 79–80, the product used in all the trials discussed in this book. A solution was prepared by mixing 15 grams of shark cartilage into

4 ounces of water. This solution was administered as a retention enema via surgical tubing attached to a large syringe. After administration, the patients lay on their left side for twenty minutes to ensure adequate absorption. Later in the study, several patients switched to oral administration. Higher doses were tried, too, and we soon discovered that the optimum dosage for a terminal cancer patient is 1 gram of shark cartilage per 2 pounds of body weight. In other words, a 180-pound man should receive 90 grams of shark cartilage per day, while a 110-pound woman should receive 55 grams per day. At these levels, we found that tumors often begin to shrink, pain decreases materially, and—when present—symptoms of rheumatoid arthritis, osteoarthritis, and psoriasis (see page 131) usually disappear quickly.

In early January 1993, eighteen patients who had remained in the study for sixteen weeks were evaluated, and the first trial was concluded. Without exception, all of the eighteen had been extremely ill when the study began. In addition, due to the economic embargo, their diets, like those of many Cubans, had long been deficient in vitamins and minerals. Despite the fact that the deck was stacked against the study, almost 40 percent of the subjects experienced significant improvement in their conditions. Furthermore, the participating physicians—both Cuban and American—agreed that even if the shark cartilage did not cure the patients, it had "dramatically improved their quality of life."

The eighteen patients evaluated were:

- An eighty-two-year-old man with prostate cancer that had metastasized to the bone. This man had been told that nothing could be done for him. After two weeks on shark cartilage, he was pain-free. After sixteen weeks, ultrasound measurements revealed that the tumor had shrunk 58 percent.

- A fifty-six-year-old man with brain cancer. In 1990, 80 percent of the tumor had been surgically removed, and the man subsequently received radiation and chemotherapy. After six weeks on shark cartilage, the subject reported feeling much better. After sixteen weeks, he had difficulty speaking, but it is highly significant that no substantial new tumor growth was detected at this time. In the majority of cases, brain tumors grow rapidly; surgery usually does not get all of the tumor, and regrowth is common.

- A seventy-three-year-old man with a fast-growing tumor at the base of his tongue. At the beginning of the study, the 30-by-32-millimeter tumor was making it impossible for the man to swallow. He had lost so much weight that he was too weak to get out of bed. After six weeks on shark cartilage, the tumor had shrunk 53 percent and the man was able to eat. At sixteen weeks, the tumor had begun to grow again.

- A seventy-two-year-old man with esophageal cancer. When he entered the program, his throat was blocked, he was in severe pain, and he was unable to eat. After four weeks, the tumor had shrunk considerably, but at sixteen weeks, it had started to grow again.

- A forty-seven-year-old woman with an extremely large ovarian tumor. At the beginning of the study, a 90-centimeter tumor filled her abdominal cavity, stretching her skin so much that movement was very painful. At six weeks, the woman was no longer in pain and ultrasound examination showed that the tumor, which had become attached to the pelvic wall, had decreased to 85 centimeters in length. At sixteen weeks, the woman was still pain-free and the tumor, which had become completely detached from the pelvic wall, was now operable. Surgical removal of the tumor is now pending.

- A forty-two-year-old woman with breast cancer that had metastasized to the lung and the liver. After seven weeks on shark cartilage, the patient reported feeling better. At that time, the tumor size was unchanged but there appeared to be changes within the tumor. This patient passed away before the sixteen-week evaluation.

- A sixty-year-old female with breast cancer that had metastasized to the bone. At sixteen weeks, a bone scan revealed possible new tumor growth.

- A sixty-three-year-old woman with ovarian cancer that had metastasized to the right lung and to the liver. X-rays at the start of the study revealed that the lung contained approximately two liters of fluid that had been produced by the tumor. Six weeks into the program, the fluid was gone. Physicians agreed that the diuretics the woman had been given could not have had that effect. It appeared that the shark cartilage aided in the removal of the fluid. The woman, however, did not survive into the sixteenth week.

- A fifty-seven-year-old woman with a breast tumor that had broken through the skin and metastasized to the lung. Although the woman had been experiencing a noticeable decrease in pain, she passed away before completing the study.

- An eighty-one-year-old woman with breast cancer that had metastasized to the bone. After six weeks of shark-cartilage therapy, the tumor had shrunk from 65 by 49 millimeters to 24 by 32 millimeters. At sixteen weeks, no further changes in the tumor were detected.

- A seventy-year-old woman with colon cancer that had metastasized to the liver. After six weeks of shark-cartilage therapy, the tumor had decreased from 33 by 49 millimeters to 24 by 32 millimeters. At sixteen weeks, all signs indicated that the liver disease had worsened.

- A sixty-three-year-old woman with breast cancer. A year after a mastectomy, the tumor had metastasized to the surgical lesion on the chest wall. After six weeks on shark-cartilage therapy, the woman was symptom-free. However, she chose to withdraw from the study.

- A forty-nine-year-old man with liver cancer that had spread to the skin. When he started taking shark cartilage, the man was in extreme pain and unable to lie down to sleep. After six weeks, he reported being free of pain, but adverse changes were detected in liver function tests. At sixteen weeks, the patient was still pain-free, but the liver appeared to have gotten larger. The physicians believe that the man's condition has improved enough so that he may now be a candidate for a liver transplant.

- A twenty-two-year-old man with nonmetastatic brain cancer. Prior to the study, a large proportion of the tumor had been surgically removed. At sixteen weeks of shark-cartilage therapy, there was no evidence of tumor regrowth.

- A fifty-nine-year-old man with brain cancer. Approximately 90 percent of the tumor had been surgically removed. Signs of intracranial pressure prompted physicians to once again operate on the man. The surgery revealed that a new tumor was growing and that a necrotic, or dead, tumor mass was also present. This mass may have necrosed because of the cartilage therapy.

- An eighteen-year-old man with brain cancer. Following surgical removal of the tumor, this patient experienced such severe equilibrium problems and muscle weakness that he was totally unable to walk. In addition, his facial nerve was paralyzed, leaving him unable to use the muscles of facial expression or to close his eyes. At the six-week evaluation, the facial paralysis had disappeared and the young man was walking and swimming. At sixteen weeks, his central nervous system problems were continuing to improve.

- A seventy-year-old man with prostatic cancer that had metastasized to the pelvic bone. X-rays taken three to four weeks after shark-cartilage therapy began revealed possible new bone formation in the area where the cancer had eroded pelvic bone. Before the sixteen-week evaluation, this patient died of an intestinal obstruction that was not related to the cancer.

- A forty-seven-year-old woman with cancer in one tonsil that had spread throughout her lymphatic system. Physicians participating in the study agreed that this patient's survival for six weeks was very significant. She passed away before the sixteen-week evaluation.

The experiences of these patients revealed five key facts:

1. The shark-cartilage product used in the study works when administered orally or rectally.

2. No intestinal bleeding or irritation occurs with oral administration of the shark-cartilage product. In some people, high oral doses cause minor gastric discomfort such as gas.

3. Rectal administration does not cause gastric discomfort nor changes in the intestinal mucosa.

4. Absolutely no toxicity was noted at any dosage level.

5. In each case, use of the shark-cartilage product significantly reduced pain. This discovery may be one of the most important findings in the study. Pain reduction seems to be the first effect of shark cartilage. It is assumed that pain is diminished because of the reduction in tumor size.

The results of the study are all the more significant when one remembers that the patients had all been considered terminal with little chance of survival using conventional cancer therapy. It's just a pity that a more exacting study could not have been done in the United States; instead, I had to turn to Cuba. Representatives of the Cuban government were so impressed by the results that a second trial will be conducted. It will involve more than 100 patients, divided into four groups of 25 according to the form of cancer with which they are stricken— breast, prostate, bone, or brain. Because I believe that patients in the first Cuban study may have experienced a plateau in tumor shrinkage due to dietary deficiencies, the second study will include the use of vitamin and mineral supplements.

AND IN NEW JERSEY

Even before the *60 Minutes* telecast, the information about shark cartilage's effect on tumors had been attracting the public's attention. Several medical doctors in my area had read an article about my work and had contacted me for more information. Interested in what I told them, these doctors began administering shark cartilage to cancer patients, monitoring their progress, and checking for side effects.

A doctor in northern New Jersey began working with patients in the summer of 1992 and soon discovered that high-level doses of shark cartilage—up to 120 grams—brought about amazing results. He has worked with more than 110 patients and has been delighted with the dramatic turnabout in their conditions. MRI and CAT scans reveal that at least 15 of this doctor's patients are basically tumor-free. Others are showing a reduction in tumor size. It is gratifying to see that there are those in the medical community who know the limitations of established cancer approaches and feel the need to provide more effective treatments.

THEORY MOVES INTO THE REAL WORLD

One of the major imports of clinical trials is that they move theory into the real world. Our trials on people have not only tested and proven the theory that shark cartilage can cause major tumor reduction but have also given us some concrete data on the method of achieving the reversal.

Although dosage data is somewhat limited, information from various trials discussed here suggests the use of high dosage levels, which is not a surprising course of action with a rapidly growing tumor. In the Jules Bordet studies, 1,200 milligrams (1.2 grams) of dry cartilage per 1 kilogram (2.2 pounds) of body weight inhibited tumor growth. This is equivalent to a 110-pound person's taking of 50 grams (about 2 ounces) daily.

High daily dosages of 50 to 60 grams are effectively administered either as retention enemas or in part as enemas and in part orally. Lower dosages given in the early stages of cancer or as a preventative measure seem to be effective when administered orally. The results of a study in Germany comparing the oral and rectal methods of administration are pending.

Since shark cartilage acts as an angiogenesis inhibitor, it is most likely to have an effect on the more heavily vascularized solid tumors. Breast, cervical, prostate, central nervous system, and pancreatic cancers are among the most heavily vascularized cancers and therefore potentially the best targets for shark-cartilage therapy. Cancers such as lymphoma, Hodgkins, and leukemia are less likely to be affected by shark cartilage since new vascularization is rarely involved in their development.

Shrinking tumors is, however, only part of shark cartilage's role in cancer control. Perhaps even more important is its potential as a prophylactic measure. Theoretically, any nontoxic natural supplement that inhibits new blood-vessel development should act as a cancer preventive at any level of use. The degree of protection is, of course, the open question. Shortly, we may have results from studies on the effects of shark cartilage as a prophylactic against cancer and other angiogenesis-dependent diseases. Hopefully, these results will help us obtain government or other major grant support for additional studies on prophylactic effects, studies that are quite costly.

MAKING USE OF THE RESEARCH RESULTS

The preventative and therapeutic effects of shark cartilage are becoming more apparent as the research continues. Preliminary findings indicate that tumors—both malignant and benign—are being reduced in size as a direct result of the administration of shark cartilage. These results are affected by route of administration (oral or rectal), by the state of the tumor (advanced or early stage), by concurrent treatments, and by the amount of shark-cartilage material used. The type of shark cartilage might also prove to be a factor. All the clinical trials that are being discussed in this book were conducted using a 100-percent-pure shark-cartilage product that is processed in accordance with the patent discussed on pages 79–80.

The data seem to indicate that with Stage III and Stage IV tumors, approximately 1 gram of shark cartilage per 2 pounds of body weight should be used on a daily basis. When possible, the material should be administered as a retention enema, but it can be administered orally if necessary. Some researchers have found that rectal administration produces the best results but that oral administration also works well. Most tumor reduction has been seen with oral/rectal administration.

Doses should be spread throughout the day to keep the level of active protein in the blood fairly constant. For example, a dose can be taken after defecating in the morning, one at bedtime, and two in between. For oral administration, mix the cartilage in a vegetable juice such as tomato, carrot, or beet juice, or in a fruit nectar. To prepare a retention enema, mix 15 grams (3 level teaspoons) of shark-cartilage powder in two-thirds of a cup of body-temperature water. Women might prefer to take at least one dose as a water suspension introduced into the vaginal cavity, especially in the case of vaginal, cervical, or uterine tumor.

Preliminary results indicate that some reduction in tumor size will be noted within six weeks after the start of treatment, and major tumor reduction will be noted within eleven weeks. When tumors are less life-threatening, the dosage level can be lowered; evidence indicates that dosage can be reduced up to 60 percent.

I want to make it crystal clear that at this time, without much more evidence, I am *not* suggesting that conventional medical approaches be replaced by shark-cartilage administration. I do believe that shark cartilage can and probably should be used along with conventional approaches. When other therapies are administered, I think the shark-cartilage dosage should remain constant until the tumors are gone.

Remember that most orthodox medical practitioners are not familiar with the work being done with shark cartilage. Patients should make decisions regarding its use—as well as the use of any therapies—based on the best information available. It's your life; it's up to you to do your homework.

Prevention of cancer is another issue. Research to determine a substance's prophylactic properties requires a long period of time as well as many case studies. However, over the past several years, I have made numerous observations regarding the use of shark cartilage to reduce the chances of metastasis development or reoccurrence of cancer. One of the most dramatic cases I observed occurred around 1988 and involved a young woman who had undergone surgery for cancer of the breast and lymph nodes. The prognosis following surgery was not good. But this bright and aggressive woman read and studied everything she could find about cancer therapy. She had read about shark cartilage, and one Sunday morning, she appeared at my front door. After questioning me extensively about the material, she begged me to supply her with some very early shark cartilage. Since then, she has taken nine capsules (just under 7 grams total) per day of shark cartilage and has encouraged many of those in a similar situation to do likewise. Although the odds of developing a reoccurrence of the cancer within two years are 30 percent, neither this woman nor any of her acquaintances has had a reoccurrence. It appears that 7 to 8 grams of shark cartilage daily may prevent reoccurrence, especially if a sound lifestyle including good nutrition is adopted and the person is of normal body weight.

THE WORK CONTINUES

Many facts and figures are now in and show that shark cartilage has a profound effect on tumors. Scientists and physicians around the world—in Texas, Germany, and New York City—are now conducting research that will expand our knowledge. Early responses with four cancer patients in Holland have already shown one case in which tumor size has been reduced by 25 percent; the remaining three cases have shown improved enzyme response and pronounced improvement in the electrical impulses from the cancerous organs.

But tumors and metastases are not the only conditions that can be controlled by shark cartilage. Once shark cartilage is in a person's system, its anti-inflammatory and antiangiogenic characteristics begin to work on a variety of diseases. Its effects on arthritis, psoriasis, and enteritis have already been demonstrated, and its probable effects on diabetic retinopathy, neovascular glaucoma, and macular degeneration have been discussed in a number of scientific journals. Many of these are "old-age" diseases, and as the mean age of the world's population continues to rise, this positive "side effect" of shark cartilage may prove to be one of its major advantages.

5.

Other Benefits

The process by which cartilage gives way to bone, allowing calcification and vascularization in the developing body, suggests a mechanism by which the body develops: it suggests that cartilage and bone include substances that profoundly affect other tissues. The idea could ultimately have major implications for the management of disease.

Arnold I. Caplan
Scientific American

Shark cartilage obviously offers tremendous potential for the prevention and cure of cancer. It appears, however, that shark cartilage can have a profound effect on a host of other conditions as well.

Dr. Patricia D'Amore and Dr. Michael Klagsbrun of Harvard Medical School and the Children's Hospital in Boston have called for studies that would teach us how to control the angiogenesis that occurs in tumor vascularization, diabetic retinopathy, and rheumatoid arthritis. Dr. Judah Folkman, whose angiogenesis hypothesis spurred much of the research discussed in this book, also believes that many disease therapies may result from angiogenesis research. In the January 1987 issue of *Science*, he questions whether the development of blood vessels in diseases such as diabetic retinopathy, rheumatoid arthritis, and cancer could be controlled by specific angiogenesis inhibitors.

Although angiogenesis is normally associated with positive body functions such as wound healing and embryonic development, there are many diseases that are caused by or dependent upon angiogenesis. Dr. Folkman has proposed that these diseases be categorized as "angiogenic diseases." Cancer, psoriasis, diabetic retinopathy, neovascular glaucoma, osteo- and rheumatoid arthritis, and inflammation are some of the most common maladies associated with angiogenesis and are therefore likely to be controlled by antiangiogenesis or, in other words, by shark cartilage.

ARTHRITIS CONTROL

While cancer annually afflicts over 1 million new victims in the United States alone, there are 70 million Americans who suffer from arthritis. About 15 percent of the world's population is afflicted with osteoarthritis, making it one of the most common chronic disorders. The lower back, arms, legs, fingers, knees, and shoulders are only some of the areas affected. Many people are almost immobilized by the disease, or by the more debilitating rheumatoid arthritis.

Rheumatoid Arthritis

Rheumatoid arthritis is an inflammatory disease primarily affecting the joints of the body. Joint defects, muscle wasting, and bone and cartilage destruction are all associated with this disorder.

Rheumatoid arthritis ranges in severity from a relatively trivial ailment that occurs once and never again, to a chronic condition that involves one or several joints, to a form that leads to complete invalidism. There are about 8 million rheumatoid arthritis sufferers in the United States who require medical attention.

Arthritis has always carried with it a pessimistic outlook; no form of medical treatment could be expected to reverse the damage. Many of those who experience only a few symptoms never go to physicians because it is generally accepted that traditional medicine cannot help very much. The main approach—and the only one that has seemed to offer relief—is the use of painkillers to alleviate the symptoms. Use of these drugs, however, may be causing a host of other health-related problems (see page 119). These problems are especially serious because the need for painkillers is probably lifelong.

Natural regression of the disease does not occur because cartilage is a tissue with one of the slowest turnover rates in the body. Surgery—complete or partial prosthetic replacement—produces the most rapid and dramatic improvements. However, it is costly, uses valuable resources, is not always totally successful, and carries an inherent risk of infection and mortality, particularly in the elderly. The risks and costs are, of course, multiplied when a patient is affected in several major joints, a common enough occurrence. It is no wonder that Dr. John Prudden writes in the Summer 1974 issue of *Seminars in Arthritis and Rheumatism*, "A material [cartilage] of such great potential benefit to so many millions of people should be made generally available as soon as possible."

Although the cause of rheumatoid arthritis is still a mystery, it is known that abnormal capillary growth can destroy joint cartilage; therefore, persistent angiogenesis appears to be at the root of the disease. Based on the association between arthritis and cartilage, Dr. Prudden conducted a study, which he described in *Seminars in Arthritis and Rheumatism*, involving nine people aged forty-three through sixty-nine who suffered from severe rheumatoid arthritis. Initially, all nine showed severe pain and stiffness, marked joint swelling, and the x-ray findings typical of the disease. Dr. Prudden found that a dose of 500 cubic centimeters (cc) of bovine cartilage subcutaneously administered for ten to thirty-five days and followed by booster doses at three- to four-week intervals as needed elicited "astonishingly good" results. The results showed that one-third of the arthritis sufferers improved from "severe" to "excellent" evaluations; the remaining two-thirds went from "severe" pain to a "good" evaluation, with the only treatment being a daily dose of cartilage.

Osteoarthritis

Osteoarthritis (OA), or osteoarthrosis, is a destructive disease of the articular cartilage, which is the cartilage in joints. This degenerative joint disease is the most prevalent rheumatic disorder affecting the musculoskeletal system; 40 million people suffer from it in the United States alone.

Osteoarthritis probably results at least in part from immune-system response. Excess pressure will cause cartilage to fragment at sites of high stress. Researchers believe that the body's immune system may interpret the fragments as injury. The body's response to the "injury" would be to generate inflammation at the site, resulting in swelling and some of the painful symptoms of osteoarthritis. (Since cartilage has no nerves, the pain experienced by the osteoarthritis patient does not arise in the cartilage.) Osteoarthritis may also begin with degeneration and thinning of the articular cartilage. Subsequent invasion of blood vessels into normally avascular cartilage then causes the cartilage to calcify.

A research paper published in 1985 in England discusses how angiogenesis speeds the destruction of cartilage because the new capillaries invade the cartilage and hurry its breakdown. This can be compared to water getting into the cracks of concrete, then freezing (which causes expansion) and breaking up the cement. If the development of new blood vessels can be inhibited, further breakdown of the cartilage can probably be arrested.

Shark cartilage appears to block the angiogenic process, and thereby significantly reduces joint inflammation and pain. These effects are achieved in part because of the large and effective amounts of mucopolysaccharides contained in shark cartilage. In almost all cases, the immobility and pain of arthritis are a result of inflammation. The inflammation-fighting mucopolysaccharides work with the angiogenesis-inhibiting proteins to produce a response that is much more significant than the response either might produce if working alone. This synergistic effect stops inflammation, pain, and further breakdown of the cartilage. Several clinical studies support these theories.

In a study conducted by Dr. John Prudden in the early 1970s and described in the Summer 1974 issue of *Seminars in Arthritis and Rheumatism*, twenty-eight arthritic patients, all with both severe pain and major functional disability, were injected with a cartilage preparation over a period of three to eight weeks. Nineteen cases showed results that were classified as "excellent"; six were considered "good"; and three were considered "fair" or to show "no response." None showed any evidence of toxicity or ill effects.

Another study using shark cartilage was conducted in 1988 by Dr. Serge Orloff, one of Western Europe's leading arthritis experts. Dr. Orloff administered dried shark cartilage to humans, giving them 9 grams of cartilage daily for four weeks followed by 4.5 grams daily for an additional, extended period. He was impressed with the results, particularly with those experienced by a forty-nine-year-old woman with femoropatellar "degenerative" joint disease and low-back pain attributable to a chronic disk condition. The woman's pain score decreased by 50 percent after the first two weeks of treatment, and then by another 50 percent after six weeks of treatment. She reported that she could bend both her knees and her back with less pain while doing her day-to-day chores and that she felt as though she had firmer muscles.

Beginning in the early 1980s, studies were conducted in five clinics in five Eastern European countries. The most significant aspect of these studies was the data on lost working days. Over a ten-year period, the patients receiving the cartilage preparation lost an average of just twenty working days per year; the patients who did not receive the cartilage preparation lost a steadily increasing number of working days, culminating in a total of 180 out of 250 by the tenth year. These "sick days," which were something the Eastern Block nations recorded faithfully, were taken primarily because of the pain associated with arthritis. The pain was decreased by 85 percent when cartilage was administered. In contrast, those patients in the control group used nonsteroidal anti-inflammatory drugs (NSAIDs) or placebos and experienced only a 5-percent reduction in pain. Joint degeneration among those using the cartilage was equal to 37 percent of the control group's joint degeneration. In a 1987 report published in *Seminars in Arthritis and Rheumatism*, V. Rejholee, M.D., concludes, "It is clear that any form of medication that is well tolerated and shown to be capable of influencing the natural history of OA, either by slowing progression or by bringing about actual regression, must be regarded as a major advance in the therapy for this condition. The implications in terms of relief of suffering, health care resources and socioeconomic costs to the community are similarly far reaching. Therefore, any therapeutic agent with indications of such activity must be considered and carefully evaluated."

Also in 1987, the results of a long-term assessment of the effects of a bovine-cartilage preparation on osteoarthritis were published by the head of the rheumatology facility at Charles University in Prague, Czechoslovakia. This was a double-blind study so that neither the 194 participating patients nor the doctors knew who was getting the cartilage material and who was getting the placebo. The pain scores in this study dropped an average of 50 percent.

In 1989, José A. Orcasita, M.D., assistant clinical professor of internal medicine at the University of Miami School of Medicine, conducted a nine-week study of six elderly victims of osteoarthritis. All of the patients had been experiencing significant pain, pain that was rated nine or ten on a scale of one to ten and that could best be described as almost unbearable. After the first visit, the patients stopped taking their prescription pain and inflammation medications and began taking the dry shark cartilage. They were evaluated weekly for nine weeks. Three of the six patients completed the nine-week course, which consisted of daily doses of 9 grams of cartilage taken orally at the rate of 3 grams three times a day, before meals. (Two of the patients left the study early, and one completed just seven-eighths of the course of treatment.) During the last five weeks of the study, the dose was cut in half but still taken in three equal doses before meals. The three patients who completed the course showed a decrease in pain of five to six points. (Even the patient who completed just seven-eighths responded well.) In all cases, a marked improvement was noted in the quality of life. Those who engaged in physical activities reported that after taking the shark cartilage, they no longer experienced pain during their activities. Dr. Orcasita said, "The patients have shown absolutely no side effects, no toxicity, no complaint of any kind."

Also in 1989, Dr. Carlos Luís Alpizar, head of the national geriatric program in Costa Rica, gave oral doses of shark cartilage to ten patients suffering from osteoarthritis so severe that they were bedridden. Within three weeks, eight of the patients were ambulatory. To ensure that the results were not due to a placebo effect—a psychological rather than a real effect—a veterinarian in Brussels, Belgium, conducted a carefully controlled study with dogs.

Research With Dogs

If you're anything like me and if you've loved a dog for a long time, you know how painful it is to watch your pet suffer. Arthritis will often turn a once-playful pup into a sedentary senior citizen, quiet at best, vicious at worst. My dog George, who at nine years of age was painfully arthritic and pitiful to see, was the first dog to whom shark-cartilage therapy was ever administered.

George received a very crude early batch of shark cartilage, given to him daily along with his food. Within two weeks, he was a new dog, back to his original active self. He lived to the age of fifteen, taking shark cartilage with food every day for the last six years of his life.

Sometimes, however, dogs don't get to live out their normal life span. Sometimes, the arthritis is so debilitating that emotionally tortured pet owners choose to put the dog "to sleep." In the hope of avoiding such an eventuality, the owners of more than a dozen dogs participated in studies conducted by Jacques Rauis, D.V.M. Dr. Rauis, a privately practicing doctor of veterinary medicine in Brussels, Belgium, and a member of the faculty of medicine at the University of Liege, reported on his study at the 1991 Small Animal Veterinary Congress in Manchester, England.

Dr. Rauis's first study was conducted with ten dogs, each of whom suffered from severe lameness. A freeze/vacuum-dried shark cartilage was used as treatment for secondary osteoarthritis. Each dog was given 750 milligrams of dry cartilage per 5 kilograms of body weight for three weeks. The cartilage powder was usually put into the dogs' meals. (Only one of the animals balked at the taste.) No other drug or food supplement or treatment was given during the test period. Each dog was evaluated according to six parameters and assigned a score between 0 and 5. The six parameters were:

   I. Local swelling; pain.
   II. Atrophy of muscles (wasting of regional muscles).
   III. Joint crepitation (the rubbing sound characteristic of osteoarthritis).
   IV. Lameness before action (difficulty walking or running after several hours of immobility).
   V. Lameness after action (difficulty walking or running after a half-hour of exercise but able to get over an obstacle not previously overcome).
   VI. Movement over obstacle (difficulty getting over an obstacle).

Table 5.1 summarizes the pre- and post-study evaluations. The dogs were evaluated at days eight, fifteen, twenty-one, and thirty-six, and again two weeks after the termination of the treatment. Dr. Rauis quickly found dramatic decreases in the signs of the disease. The animals' lameness disappeared, and their capacity for getting around obstacles improved tremendously. Swelling, pain, and immobilization were negligible. Only two of the dogs did not show these dramatic results. The owners of the other dogs reported that their pets were more alert, jumped "as never before," were "much more alive" and "very happy," and were "able to climb the stairs alone." One even referred to the results as "spectacular." The only side effect reported was the increased appetite evidenced by Ada, a seven-year-old female Labrador.

In all cases, when the cartilage was discontinued after day twenty-one, the dogs reverted in large part to their original pained state within fifteen days. When the shark cartilage was again added to the diet, the improvement seemed to be even

Table 5.1.   Scores of Arthritic Dogs
Before and After Treatment With Shark Cartilage

	I Local Swelling; Pain	II Atrophy of Muscles	III Joint Crepitation	IV Lameness Before Action	V Lameness After Action	VI Movement Over Obstacle
Test Dog 1	5/3	2/2	4/2	3/1	3/1	5/4
Test Dog 2	3/1	3/3	4/3	5/3	5/3	5/3
Test Dog 3	3/0	1/1	1/1	2/0	2/1	4/2
Test Dog 4	3/0	3/3	3/3	3/2	4/2	5/1
Test Dog 5	1/1	0/0	3/2	3/2	2/1	3/2
Test Dog 7	1/0	1/1	3/0	2/2	3/2	3/2
Test Dog 8	3/0	3/3	4/2	5/1	4/2	5/3
Test Dog 9	3/1	3/3	3/3	3/2	3/2	4/2
Test Dog 10	1/1	2/2	3/3	3/2	2/2	3/3
Test Dog 11	4/2	2/1	2/2	2/1	2/1	4/2

The scores on the left are the result of testing before administration of shark cartilage. A score of 0 is the best and a score of 5 is the worst.

Test Dog 6 was withdrawn from the study.

better and quicker than the original response. This improvement was achieved with 50 percent of the original dosage level.

Dr. Rauis's observation was that the main effect seemed to be against the local swelling. In addition, he felt that the effect on the functional signs was "also impressive." His summation: "Shark cartilage in this preliminary report appears both effective and safe to administer in the treatment of canine osteoarthritis."

Dr. Rauis subsequently studied another six dogs with similar results.

Ben B. Dow, D.V.M., who has a private practice in Vermont, has been administering shark cartilage to arthritic older dogs in his care. He recently wrote to me, saying, "I am using the shark cartilage product and after 25 years as a practitioner I have to admit that the results are better than with all the other drugs we have at our disposal to treat arthritis. All the steroids have many side effects which are sometimes worse than the condition itself."

Dr. Dow goes on in his letter to detail the successful treatment of a nine-year-old Golden Labrador whose arthritis was so severe, "the dog refused to get in and out of a vehicle or go up or down stairs." Although the owners were ready to put the dog to sleep, the animal is now jumping from the ground into a pickup truck and playing Frisbee. With this animal as well as the others treated by Dr. Dow, "It took no more than three weeks for a drastic change to occur. . . . There were also no side effects that were undesirable."

The dog studies confirm the results that have been achieved in humans and eliminate the possibility of the effect's being psychological rather than physiological. These results indicate shark cartilage is a completely safe nontoxic natural product that can alleviate the pain of arthritis. The importance of such a product cannot be overemphasized, given the serious side effects of medications currently used in the treatment of arthritis. (The only "side effect" of shark cartilage is its potential for preventing serious maladies.)

Panama Studies Confirm Earlier Work

In Panama, Harry Xatrush, M.D., has also been investigating the effects of shark cartilage on arthritis. In one clinical trial, a man with a painful condition in the spinal column and in the muscles of the back and hip began receiving shark-cartilage capsules in September 1990. He had suffered with the painful condition for five years, and different specialists had offered different diagnoses including osteoarthritis. His symptoms included pain upon moving, severe morning stiffness, and cramps in the muscles of the back.

The daily dosage for this condition was one capsule of cartilage per every 11 pounds of body weight. After eighteen days, the morning stiffness and muscular cramps had been eliminated. By the fifth week, all the symptoms had disappeared.

Another clinical trial involved a forty-two-year-old man

with a painful chronic inflammatory illness that had been diagnosed in 1966 as rheumatoid arthritis. Since that time, the patient had been treated with a variety of medications including analgesics, salicylates, nonsteroidal anti-inflammatory drugs, gold salts, immunosupressants, and corticoids. These medications had produced a variety of side effects "without controlling the disease in any satisfactory way."

In January 1991, when the patient began receiving shark-cartilage capsules, he was a bedridden invalid with intense pain and deformity in the large joints. The course of his treatment consisted of one capsule per 11 pounds of body weight for twenty-one days, then four capsules per day for the next twenty-one days. After three weeks of treating the patient, investigators noted that his spinal column had straightened and his pain had completely disappeared. The patient now says, "My spine has straightened out; I am able to move my arms and legs without pain; my walk has improved; I am more agile. I feel like working; I'm not tired and my constipation and gastritis have improved." He continues to take four capsules of the shark-cartilage product along with 5 milligrams of prednisone and sulindac in isolated form every forty-eight hours.

Eliminating Adverse Side Effects

Not only is shark cartilage effective against arthritis, but it is largely inert and nontoxic and therefore can usually be used in conjunction with other therapies. Cartilage's modes of action—namely, stimulation of the immune system and inhibition of a new blood network—should not interfere with other therapies, no matter how drastic or simple the chosen therapy. More importantly, shark cartilage has none of the adverse side effects of the most commonly used medications.

Recent statistics have shown that elderly people, who are

most often the victims of arthritis, are the most likely to suffer from the complications related to the drugs generally used for arthritic conditions. In one study of an elderly Medicaid population, physicians found that those people who used prescription nonsteroidal anti-inflammatory drugs (NSAIDs) were more than *four times* as likely to die from peptic ulcer or upper gastrointestinal hemorrhage than were nonusers.

NSAIDs—eiflunisal, profen, ibuprofen, indomethacin, salicylate, and tolmetin—are currently the most commonly prescribed medications for arthritis sufferers. Because of this, even small risks may have major public-health implications. We now know that the risks of NSAID use are anything but small.

It has long been known that aspirin can cause peptic ulcers and plays a role in duodenal ulcers, but the role of nonaspirin NSAIDs in peptic ulcers has been controversial. Current research does, however, indicate a causal association between NSAIDs and fatal peptic ulcers, revealing that 29 percent of the fatalities can be attributed to the drugs. NSAIDs increase the risk of clinically serious peptic ulcers, particularly for the elderly.

There is a $2 billion market for NSAIDs worldwide, and more than 70 million prescriptions were written in the United States alone in a single year in the late 1980s. Arthritis patients use between twenty and twenty-four NSAID pills daily, day in and day out. Although NSAIDs had been considered safe, the Arthritis Advisory Committee of the Food and Drug Administration has, since 1988, been calling for new labeling for these drugs, labeling that would caution users of the risks of ulceration, bleeding, and perforation. A chief danger for NSAID users is that the intestinal lining can be injured without the appearance of any obvious symptoms. This means that serious consequences can occur without warning signs. People have actually fainted from excessive blood loss without having seen any signs of trouble. Patients with previous stomach disorders or debilitating diseases as well as the elderly appear to be the most susceptible to these gastric complications.

Shark Cartilage Is a Viable Alternative

Thousands of Americans die each year of NSAID-related hemorrhages. Hundreds of millions of dollars are spent on health care and lost productivity. No wonder many practitioners and researchers are calling for further studies to determine which drugs and/or dosages might be less toxic. An editorial in the September 1, 1988, issue of *Annals of Internal Medicine* calls for testing to determine a more realistic approach to this pervasive therapy. The testing would itself involve significant expense—expense that would be passed on to the consumer—and would require several years to complete. Such testing may not be necessary in light of the findings that shark cartilage is completely safe and nontoxic as well as effective.

Shark cartilage is available today as a food supplement, and researchers have found that shark cartilage is successful in reducing pain in approximately 70 percent of osteoarthritis cases and 60 percent of rheumatoid arthritis cases. Experience to date suggests that the pain of arthritis can be alleviated through the use of 1 gram of dried shark cartilage for every 15 pounds of body weight (or one 740- to 750-milligram capsule per 11 pounds of body weight) taken daily for approximately twenty-one days. Investigators have found this dosage to be most effective when divided into three equal doses, each taken about fifteen minutes before a meal. Generally speaking, users experience pain relief within sixteen to eighteen days when the shark cartilage is used regularly. If major pain relief is not observed after thirty days of continuous and correct use, the cartilage will probably not work with your system or problem. Positive responses are easily recognized.

Once pain relief is noted, investigators decrease the dosage level to 1 gram for each 40 pounds of body weight (or one 740- to 750-milligram capsule per 30 pounds of body weight). The maintenance dosage may be consumed all at once or divided into two equal doses, depending on the preference of the user.

Pain will probably not be completely eliminated, but it will be significantly reduced. When the use of shark cartilage is discontinued for two weeks, the pain normally returns to the same level of severity as before treatment started.

Arthritis is not the only angiogenesis-dependent disease for which shark cartilage may be an efficacious therapy. In several studies concentrating on arthritis patients, fortuitous side effects were discovered. Patients who suffered from eczema in addition to arthritis noted improvement in the skin condition. Subsequent research demonstrated that shark cartilage is indeed effective against skin diseases such as psoriasis, poison oak and ivy, and acne.

PSORIASIS AND OTHER SKIN CONDITIONS

Psoriasis affects millions of people, most commonly and persistently on the scalp, elbows, and knees but also on the entire body. Psoriasis is characterized by excessive growth and shedding of the outer layer of skin. The condition may depend on abnormal capillary growth in the skin, resulting in unusually large increases in skin thickness above the capillary bed. Treatment of psoriasis generally involves corticosteroid creams and ointments, coal tar preparations, and ultraviolet light. In extreme cases, methotrexate—a drug that may damage the liver—is used. The response to these therapies is erratic and in most cases must be considered poor. Far superior results were obtained by Dr. Prudden, according to his scientific report in the Summer 1974 issue of *Seminars in Arthritis and Rheumatism*, which included a discussion of a successful treatment of thirty-nine patients.

Dr. Prudden discovered cartilage's potential as a psoriasis therapy by chance during treatment of a nonhealing ulcer on the leg of a man who also had psoriasis. Dr. Prudden had long been using cartilage preparations to accelerate wound healing; with this purpose in mind, he applied a preparation of cartilage powder to the cleaned ulcer. The leg was wrapped with a dressing and then bandaged. When the dressing was removed three days later, the ulcer—which went on to heal completely—had improved as expected. In addition, the psoriasis had significantly improved. According to Dr. Prudden, the dressing had closed off the area, trapping the cartilage, which was then spread about by the fluid escaping from the ulcer.

To confirm his findings regarding cartilage's effects on psoriasis, Dr. Prudden administered injections of Catrix-S, a cartilage product prepared especially for subcutaneous administration, to thirty-nine people who had psoriasis on up to 70 percent of their bodies. Of these cases, nineteen experienced total remission; lesions disappeared for six weeks to more than one year. The average length of remission—characterized by a rather rapid descaling—was approximately five months. The skin turned smooth, but the dilated capillary bed remained undiminished. With continued treatment, this capillary network "shut down" and the skin returned to normal.

Of the sixteen patients who did not experience a complete remission within two months, fifteen still had good results; only one had poor results. Dr. Prudden considered this variation to be due to the psychology of psoriatic patients. Patients with psoriasis are often quite pessimistic about the possibility of a cure. Those who consent to experimental therapies have probably suffered excessively and already tried many treatments unsuccessfully. Their consent, however, indicates their strong hope that cure is possible. This combination of what Prudden calls "mystic faith and profound skepticism" is what makes it difficult to ensure consistent treatment and follow-up.

In addition, of the sixteen patients who did not achieve remission with the series of injections, eleven went into complete remission after additional treatments of booster 50-cc injections of Catrix-S every three weeks and topical application of 5-percent Catrix ointment. The ointment, which is applied twice a day after bathing or three times a day if practical for the patient, need not be accompanied by wrapping. When the lesions were elevated, dry, and horny, a cartilage preparation with 0.1 percent coal tar, USP (prepared as specified in the United States Pharmacopia), led to more rapid descaling. Once the lesions were smooth and red, an ointment without coal tar was used. With this therapy regimen, booster injections were usually not necessary. Even in this more difficult group, the remissions lasted from ten to fourteen months before repeat therapy was necessary.

Of the remaining cases, Dr. Prudden writes in his scientific article, "Because of increased confidence in the efficacy of the topical Catrix preparations following the formulation adjustments . . . and because we did not realize that the parenteral dose [dose by injection] must be increased to at least 1500 cc if a satisfactory response is not achieved at lower dose ranges . . . we are confident that we can produce remissions in these individuals as well."

In the same article, Dr. Prudden reports that a number of patients were also treated successfully for poison oak and poison ivy. The first to be treated was a forty-one-year-old woman who had gone to gather "beautiful red leaves." She gathered more than she had bargained for, developing a severe case of poison oak that spread all over her hands, arms, legs, and face. "Maddening" itch, edema (the presence of large amounts of fluid in the intercellular tissue spaces), and peeling skin were combined with swelling that increased the size of her face and arms more than one and a half times their norm. Despite applications of various prescription creams, the itching interfered with the woman's sleep. Her incessant scratching was beginning to cause secondary infections. Treated with 5-percent Catrix cream, the woman reported relief within five minutes. Within two weeks, her skin returned to normal.

Dr. Prudden also reported treating an additional six cases of severe poison ivy in which the lesions cleared in about a week. The itching was controlled for increasingly long periods of time whenever the cartilage preparation was applied. Again, no relief had been obtained with topical corticosteroids.

Finally, in two other studies, the cartilage preparation's

potential for preventing allergic reaction was investigated. In one of the studies, one forearm of a volunteer was spread with the Catrix cream, while the other forearm was spread with only the cream base. The volunteer then walked into poison ivy. No reaction was evident on the treated arm, but the other arm showed typical allergic reactions.

Other "skin" conditions successfully treated with a cartilage preparation include acne; mandibular alveolitis ("dry socket"), an extremely painful gum condition that sometimes follows tooth extractions; and pruritus ani, intense chronic itching in the anal area. In addition, suppositories prepared from bovine cartilage were successfully used to treat hemorrhoids.

While most of the reports on psoriasis and other skin disorders are based on work done with a bovine-cartilage preparation, one should remember that *research at MIT found shark cartilage to be 1,000 times more effective than bovine cartilage as an angiogenesis inhibitor* (see page 45). In addition, significantly similar responses have been seen in people who used shark cartilage to reduce inflammation. The logical conclusion then is that the results published for bovine cartilage can be duplicated with shark cartilage. In fact, Dr. Jergen Oberle, a medical doctor in Dusseldorf, Germany, reported in May 1992 on three advanced psoriasis patients treated with shark cartilage taken orally and applied as a 10-percent topical ointment. All three patients responded favorably after four to six weeks of treatment. Shark cartilage also has more of the angiogenesis-inhibiting factor than bovine cartilage, which means that users of shark cartilage may get the added bonus of prevention of other serious diseases.

Most recently, J. J. Hernandez-Pombo, M.D., a Florida-based physician, used shark cartilage for one of his patients. The woman had suffered from psoriasis for twenty-five years and had found little relief through conventional psoriasis treatments such as cortisone and coal tar. Dr. Pombo administered 15 grams of shark cartilage per day, and after just eight days, there was a 50-percent improvement in the woman's condition.

Experience is limited but already indicates that the effective dosage level for psoriasis is 15–25 grams daily depending on body weight. Be aware that with this treatment, the itching and scales will be the first symptoms to disappear. Without the scales, the redness of the skin will appear to intensify since the large bed of capillary vessels will be more apparent. This capillary bed will also slowly disappear over a period of sixty to ninety days.

ENTERITIS

Cartilage has also been successfully used by Dr. Prudden to treat regional enteritis, an inflammation in the lining of the bowels. Although the patients had not been restored to complete health at the time Dr. Prudden wrote his scientific report for the Summer 1974 issue of *Seminars in Arthritis and Rheumatism*, they were gaining weight, strength, and optimism. Furthermore, in a 1991 study in southern California at the Comprehensive Medical Clinic, two patients with candida enteritis responded quickly to shark cartilage administered orally at the rate of 9 grams per day.

The administration of shark cartilage has yielded very good response with all sorts of intestinal inflammation. A doctor on the West Coast once told me that he advised many of his patients with intestinal inflammation to use shark cartilage as a food supplement. The doctor had been treating these patients with chondroitin sulfate, a mucopolysaccharide, but he had had success in only about half the cases. Chondroitin sulfate is cheap, but the doctor found that it doesn't seem to perform in difficult cases. When the doctor began to administer shark cartilage, he saw improvement in 80 to 90 percent of the more difficult cases.

According to the doctor, the dosage that brought about the good results is 1 gram per 15 pounds of body weight taken daily until the condition improves. Improvement usually occurred in less than thirty days. The dosage was always divided into three equal parts, each taken approximately fifteen minutes before a meal.

BLINDNESS

Although I am just now pulling together the people to undertake a formal study of the effects of shark cartilage on blindness, many researchers feel the results are a foregone conclusion. This is because many types of blindness are caused by angiogenesis. Diabetic retinopathy, macular degeneration, and venous occlusion in the retinal circulatory system are a few of the ocular disorders characterized by the growth of new retinal blood vessels. Apparently, under normal conditions, stringent mechanisms operate to prevent the growth of microvessels. During disease onset, these mechanisms are somehow overridden so that neovascularization occurs.

In diabetics, for instance, the small blood vessels that transverse the retina dilate and develop small ruptures. These ruptures leave residues that usually impede vision. New blood vessels begin to form and extend throughout the injured portion of the eye, also interfering with vision. Called diabetic retinopathy, this is currently one of the common causes of blindness.

Macular Degeneration

In American adults over the age of sixty-five, age-related macular degeneration is the most common cause of irreversible blindness. Macular degeneration is deterioration of the macula lutea, an area of the retina near the optic nerve that is essential for accurate sight. In one type of macular degeneration—exudative or wet—the degeneration begins with a proliferation of blood vessels that leak under the central portion of the retina, causing damage and scarring that eventually lead to blindness. No one knows why the blood vessels begin to proliferate. It is known, however, that early detection and removal of the leaking vessels is crucial. The light-detecting macular cells cannot recover after the leaking blood has done its damage.

Currently, in cases of exudative macular degeneration, lasers are used to cauterize the new blood vessels during the early stages of the disease, thereby preventing the retinal architecture from being disrupted. Such treatment, however, is effective in only about 25 percent of all cases. The difficulty lies in aiming the laser beam precisely enough to destroy only the abnormal vessels. Even if each "hit" is correct, a "score" still destroys a portion of the retina, thereby adversely affecting vision. The procedure is also very costly and must be repeated frequently as new vessels continue to appear. The use of a safe, inexpensive nontoxic product like shark cartilage would certainly be preferable.

Although there is no data at this time, researchers believe that the same dosage that works for psoriasis should prevent such eye disorders as exudative macular degeneration, diabetic retinopathy, and neovascular glaucoma (increased pressure in the eyeball caused by angiogenesis). In other words, 1 gram of shark cartilage per 15 pounds of body weight should act prophylactically, eliminating vessels before they develop.

AN IMPORTANT CONSIDERATION

It is important to remember that no matter how safe a product is, there are times when that product should not be used. A person who recently suffered a heart attack, for instance, needs to rebuild blood vessels. Such a person should not use an angiogenesis inhibitor for at least three months or as advised by his or her physician. (Angiogenesis during healing would probably be complete in approximately thirty days, which is considered to be the body's natural repair period.) A pregnant woman who is building a blood network to feed the developing embryo should not use shark cartilage. Women who are attempting to conceive should also avoid taking shark cartilage, which may interfere with vascularization during the menstrual cycle. Also, people who have recently had deep surgery and therefore need new blood vessels to speed healing should not use shark cartilage, nor should people involved in a major muscle-building program. Since children's blood vessels are still developing, careful consideration should be given to their use of angiogenesis inhibitors.

Blood-vessel cells have been shown to have a very long life; they are rarely replaced. Only diseases that require a new blood network cause neovascularization. This means that if you deny the new network its nourishment, you will, hopefully, prevent the disease from ever developing. The side effects of prolonged inhibition of capillary growth in healthy adults are unknown, however. It appears that delayed wound healing and contraception may be among the few detectable side effects of therapy lasting eight weeks or more.

ANTIANGIOGENESIS IS LAUDED
BY THE SCIENTIFIC COMMUNITY

All of the research discussed in this book implies that the development of angiogenesis inhibitors may solve many of today's most pressing health problems. And this book is not alone in that belief. Just consider the following headline from the June 1981 issue of *Science:*

ANGIOGENESIS INHIBITORS LINK MANY DISEASES

A new class of compounds that block
blood vessel proliferation may provide
therapy for diseases as diverse
as cancer and diabetic retinopathy

This same article, by Thomas H. Maugh III, reports, "Angiogenesis inhibition is by now a well-documented and fairly common phenomenon." Yet, since the article was published, no angiogenesis inhibitors except shark cartilage have been made commercially available. Maugh points out, "Purification and characterization of the inhibitors has, in fact, been the major bottleneck in angiogenesis studies."

Is Nero fiddling while Rome burns? Are people dying, suffering pain or limb deformity, or going blind while researchers attempt to purify the inhibitors found in shark cartilage? The evidence presented here indicates that shark cartilage—a naturally occurring substance that does not require purification—can already, as Maugh says, "provide therapy for diseases as diverse as cancer and diabetic retinopathy."

Conclusion

*It is not the disease but neglect of the remedy
which generally destroys life.*

From the Latin

As it becomes increasingly apparent that shark-cartilage therapy can be used to treat a host of diseases, I am becoming aware that this may seem like an ecological disaster for sharks. There is some fear that the use of shark cartilage may endanger the survival of the shark. Let us, however, remember that *sharks are being killed at this very moment.*

Each year, an estimated 5 to 7 million sharks are caught, killed, "de-finned," and thrown back into the water. This practice has been growing modestly for at least fifteen years.

The tuna fleet is responsible for much of the "fin-fishing." After removing the fins, the tuna fishermen discard about 90 percent of the sharks they killed. This is a terrible waste of nutritious meat and of cartilage, two most valuable resources.

Consider, too, that when sharks are believed to be a nuisance to fishermen or a threat to their lives instead of an asset to their livelihoods, wholesale slaughter of sharks often results. According to Jack Casey, the marine scientist rumored to be the inspiration for the character of Matt Hooper in *Jaws*, "Thirty years ago people would kill sharks because they thought that every dead shark meant more gamefish in the sea."

There is certainly a need to prevent overfishing; the shark is a slow-growing creature that requires sufficient time to mature and breed. Human beings—almost the only natural predators of the shark—must use their intelligence to preserve this animal. We have the ability and the responsibility to do so. But the real need is for better utilization of sharks as a valuable resource.

Thomas H. Lineaweaver III and Richard H. Backus, authors of *The Natural History of Sharks*, try to assuage the fears about overfishing by writing, "A sea fishery has yet to threaten a sea fish with extinction. The point may be reached where a particular stock of fish becomes so depleted as to make further exploitation unprofitable. But that point is reached before the stock is too depleted to renew itself sooner or later. This is not to speak in behalf of unbridled fishing; it is to say that in the long run, the fishery suffers more from overfishing, given the present state of the art, than does the fish."

Although sharks roam widely, many of them are territorial in nature, which means that heavy fishing in any one area can deplete a local population. The worldwide population is in an acceptable state, especially the population in the Indian Ocean, which is slightly warmer than the other oceans, and the zone around the equator. These two areas are home to the majority of the world's sharks. The institution of regulations to preserve local shark populations is important, but greater utilization of the animal instead of haphazard killing for fins alone is the real key to the shark's survival, especially if the potential for shark cartilage as a health product develops as it logically should.

THE PROMISE OF SHARK CARTILAGE

The promise of a cure for cancer has burst upon us before—like fireworks in a night sky. Radiation therapy, laetrile, and interferon all held promises that were not fulfilled. Will shark cartilage be counted among them in the annals of medicine?

The evidence seems to say otherwise.

Shark cartilage is already being used routinely in skin grafts for burn victims (see page 33); it is particularly useful in this area because it is not rejected by the human body. And in the past twenty years, there has been no more dramatic response with terminal cancer patients than that achieved with shark cartilage. Nothing approaches it. Yet, in conventional medicine, anything that shows a 3- or 4-percent positive result is labeled a "breakthrough." Unfortunately, with the drugs that have netted this response rate, the level of toxicity can also kill the patient. But, these are the drugs that get "good press," while shark cartilage remains a "secret."

Although angiogenesis and its effects on tumors have been well known for more than twenty years, only a handful of practitioners of alternative and complementary therapies are today using shark cartilage to treat patients with cancer. (The names of physicians who use shark-cartilage therapy can be found in John M. Fink's *Third Opinion*, which is listed in the bibliography at the end of this book.) Despite their debilitating side effects, surgery, chemotherapy, and radiation are still the most commonly used treatments. (See "Importation of Unapproved Drugs for Personal Use" on page 140.) And while scores of people die and scores more suffer from the effects of traditional therapies, scientists continue to believe that identification, purification, and synthesis of the protein(s) responsible for

Importation of Unapproved Drugs for Personal Use

For many years, the FDA has had guidelines that allow district offices to exercise discretion when determining whether or not to allow entry, for personal use only, of drugs sold abroad but not approved in the United States. When permission is granted, the petitioner may import just enough of the drug for up to three months' personal use. Several unapproved drugs that some consider of therapeutic benefit for AIDS and AIDS-related conditions have thus been allowed entry into the country.

People usually bring such products into the country in their baggage when they return from abroad. These drugs may also be imported by mail. The FDA's policy on mail importation as of December 11, 1989, is that if there is no evidence of unreasonable risk, fraud, or promotion, permissive discretion may be applied and the product mailed providing:

- *The product was purchased for personal use.*

- *The product is not for commercial distribution, and the amount of the product is not excessive (i.e., there is just enough for up to three months' use).*

- *The intended use of the product is appropriately identified.*

- *The patient seeking to import the product affirms in writing that it is for his or her own use and provides the name and address of the licensed physician in the United States who is responsible for directing the treatment with the product.*

If the imported product is considered fraudulent or dangerous, or if it is promoted for use in the United States despite a lack of approval, the FDA issues "import alerts." Up to July 27, 1988, there were forty import alerts restricting entry of medical products considered fraudulent or unsafe. These restricted products included laetrile, Immuno-Augmentative Therapy agents, and products promoted by Dr. Hans Nieper of West Germany. On January 27, 1992, the FDA issued Import Alert Number 66-57: "Automatic Detention of Foreign Manufactured Unapproved Prescription Drugs Promoted to Individuals in the U.S." This alert lists some firms that have products on automatic detention because of promotional activities.

The latest information on the FDA's policy on importing drugs can be obtained from local FDA offices or by writing to:

United States Department of Health
and Human Services
Public Health Service
Food and Drug Administration (HFI-35)
5600 Fishers Lane
Rockville, MD 20857

angiogenesis is the only way to go. Nothing could be further from the truth.

Proteins are easily denatured by heat, various chemicals, and other manufacturing processes. The problem can perhaps be best explained by using the common egg. The white of an egg, the albumen protein, is soluble in water until it is heated. Heat causes it to coagulate. When it coagulates, it changes from colorless to white, from liquid to solid, from water soluble to water insoluble. The egg protein is still the same protein, but it has been materially changed. Its chemical analysis is the same, but its biological activity and appearance are completely different.

A change in activity and appearance is only part of the problem involved in synthesis. The fact is that isolation removes the protein from its environment. In the case of shark cartilage, isolating the angiogenesis-inhibiting protein would mean separating it from the mucopolysaccharide that has the anti-inflammatory effect. Would the resulting substance be as effective? And can any of the several proteins responsible for inhibition of angiogenesis be separated from the others without changing its efficacy? (We know that there are at least three proteins responsible for the antiangiogenesis effect.) How long will it take to find out? Another twenty years? How many people will develop degenerative diseases while the investigation continues? How many will die while a nonchemical, natural, whole product could be saving lives?

FACING DOWN BIG BUSINESS

Changing the status quo is difficult, if not impossible, even with the best product or procedure. In many stories of disease control, "solving the mystery" shakes cherished beliefs and puts a lot of people out of business. The Salk Vaccine is a perfect example (see page 90).

Orthodox medicine's reaction to the use of shark cartilage sometimes brings to mind scientists of yesterday—men like Galileo, Pasteur, and Lister, who were scorned, ostracized, or excommunicated when their investigations broke with the accepted wisdom of the times. More recent but no less telling is the case of Henry Heimlich, M.D., the man who developed the Heimlich maneuver, which has already saved the lives of more than 35,000 choking Americans. This procedure—incredibly good and simple—had been, according to Dr. Heimlich, ridiculed and suppressed for ten maceutical industries.

We are all keenly aware of how health-care costs have
skyrocketed. To each of us, this is a "pain in the pocket," but
it's also more. It's an indication that health care is the fastest
growing and *most profitable* industry in the United States today.
People's lives are sometimes forfeited because they cannot
afford decent care, but the health-care industry goes on charg-
ing megabucks, which we continue to fork over.

An estimated $700 billion is spent annually in the United
States alone on pharmaceuticals, doctors, hospitals, clinics,
therapy, health foods, and auxiliary services such as ambu-
lances and invalid transportation. Just imagine the pressure
groups that become involved when a relatively low-cost item
aimed at preventing some of mankind's major diseases is presented. Think of the money those diseases represent!

A loss of income—directly or through pressure from the
pharmaceutical industry—may be one of the reasons that government agencies resist conducting or funding research into
natural products such as shark cartilage. Each year, the National Cancer Institute spends more than $1 billion on research
in its own facilities and on outside research at universities and
other centers—more than $1 billion *from our taxes*. But this
organization has consistently refused to fund research into or
to investigate natural products except in token amounts.

It pains me to see so many "good" scientists who seem to
be more interested in money and peer acceptance than in doing
good for the common man. The common man is, after all,
paying the research bills with his tax dollars. Of course, I'm
oversimplifying a bit. Researchers need to earn a living just like

the rest of us do, and many of them have learned—sometimes the hard way—that the only way to succeed is to "play the game by the rules." They know that they won't get funding or jobs—and ultimately won't be able to do any research—unless they pursue the research paths that are acceptable. And just what is the "acceptable research path"? Purification, isolation, and synthesis.

A 1984 issue of *Scientific American* reveals just how "natural" it is for scientists to think in these "chemical" terms. In the article "Cartilage," Dr. Arnold Caplan writes, "The substance [an angiogenesis inhibitor] is well worth finding, if only because the growth of a tumor requires a rich supply of blood. Perhaps a factor derived from cartilage, applied to a growing tumor, could throttle its blood supply and thus bring on its death. In any event, the search for the substance exemplifies the activity at a number of universities and corporations. Programs at these institutions are directed at isolating and purifying from adult cartilage several substances that may turn out to affect many aspects of growth, development and disease."

Why is so much effort going into "isolating and purifying" a substance *from* cartilage? Why aren't researchers and practitioners utilizing dry, whole natural shark cartilage? The answer probably combines both narrow vision and the profit motive.

Because the FDA does not sanction natural products, organizations such as NIH are reluctant to fund research on such products. This automatically rules out research on products that are not processed in a chemically pure form. Such "chemicalization" often opens the doors to toxicity, side effects, and a high cost for consumers. Someone has to pay for securing FDA approval, a process that can take up to twenty years and that costs approximately $231 million as determined by a recent Tufts University study.

There is a danger that the orthodox scientists will continue to attempt a synthesis instead of testing the potential of whole shark cartilage, a danger that might result in loss of life—over half a million people die from cancer each year in the United States. We must be alert to this danger so as to prevent its becoming an actuality. A cancer cure may put a lot of people out of work—health-care professionals, researchers, government bureaucrats. Are there individuals who will therefore attempt to squash a cure or keep it dangling like a carrot in front of the public rather than release it to save lives? Are there those in the pharmaceutical industry who would squash a natural product in order to ensure that the synthesized product will corner the market? Just think of baby formula—how much more common is its use than the use of mother's milk, a whole, natural product if ever there was one? Manufacturers of formula push its use even in Third World countries, where the women can so ill afford to spend the money. These are questions we must ask ourselves because only our awareness can protect us. (See "The Consumer's Role in the FDA" on page 146.)

STRENGTH IN NUMBERS

Awareness is only half of the picture; the other half is unity. If we stand back and look at the situation, we can see that when individuals join together, they can make a difference. Consider the case of AIDS.

As the number of AIDS fatalities mounted, scores of grieving brothers and sisters, fathers and mothers, husbands and wives, were left with nothing but their pain and their loss. They were being told by the government, "We'll get to it when we get to it. These are the procedures, the rules we must follow." What a callous answer to people in pain!

And government officials knew that the incidence of AIDS was increasing. Ever-increasing numbers of people would suffer.

And so the AIDS people—the ill, their friends, and the bereaved—got together. They formed groups that said, "This is

The Consumer's Role in the FDA

"Complacent" sometimes seems like a synonym for "consumer." Perhaps because consumers often feel powerless, they tend to accept whatever is given them. When it comes to the FDA, however, consumers do have power.

It is the "expressed wish of the FDA" for consumers to voice their needs, opinions, and desires so that these can be considered when rules, policies, or programs are put into operation. In order for the consumer to participate fully, the FDA publicizes its proposed regulations and holds public meetings to discuss the proposals. Before the FDA can establish, amend, or repeal any rule or regulation, it must—by law—publish its intentions in the "Federal Register," which is usually available at public libraries and local United States congressional offices. The notices section of the "Federal Register" includes information about hearings, investigations, and committee meetings. It also has notices of intent, which state the FDA's intention to develop a proposal to change a regulation or issue a new one, and invite public comment. Public meetings or briefings that will explain significant issues are also listed. Occasionally, however, there are legal constraints that prohibit comments from the general public, as during a hearing before a public board of inquiry when only evidence on the record may be presented.

In addition, any individual, consumer group, or industry group can petition the commissioner of the FDA "to initiate, change or revoke a regulation." The petitioner should write to the commissioner, stating the problem and proposing specific action.

To keep up-to-date, consumers should periodically review the "Federal Register" or subscribe to the "FDA Consumer," the agency's official magazine. Subscriptions to both can be obtained from the Superintendent of Documents, Washington, DC 20402, or copies can be reviewed at local FDA offices.

Consumers who do get involved can make a difference. In recent years, AIDS activists have pressured the FDA into changing its policies to allow the rapid distribution of any drugs that may be effective against AIDS so that lives may be prolonged. In March 1987, these activists secured approval of AZT for AIDS treatment. AZT (zidovudine, formerly called azidothymidine) was rushed through the FDA testing process in a record time of just over two years. The FDA normally requires animal studies of one to two years followed by clinical trials that can take from two to ten years to complete. The FDA then reviews the evidence from the trials for an additional two months to seven years. All in all, it takes a new drug four to twenty years to get into the marketplace.

The outcries by AIDS patients demanding access to experimental drugs also helped convince President George Bush to convene a committee to investigate possible changes in FDA procedures. At a public meeting in February 1989, the committee considered how federal researchers and regulatory agencies could quickly get experimental drugs to patients dying of AIDS and cancer while ensuring drug safety and effectiveness. The head of the panel, Louis Lasagna, M.D., then dean of Tufts Medical School, said, "There's a tendency for the public to favor a more libertarian point of view today. They're saying, 'I don't want Big Daddy to make judgments for me' . . . The patient should be the judge not the FDA."

Dr. Lasagna and the National Committee to Review Current Procedures for Approval of New Drugs for Cancer and AIDS submitted their final report on August 15, 1990. Included

*was an eight-point summary of the twenty-six-page report.
Among the points were:*

> II. *The Need for More and Better Drugs for Cancer
> and AIDS. A national policy should be adopted
> to foster the development of new drugs for AIDS
> and cancer in order to meet the needs for all
> patients who suffer from these diseases . . .*
>
> III. *Expediting Approval of Important New Drugs.
> The FDA should continue to exercise its statu-
> tory and administrative flexibility to approve
> AIDS and cancer drugs for marketing at the
> earliest possible point in their development . . .*
>
> XVI. *The Expanded Access (Parallel Track) IND
> [Investigational New Drug]. Where there is
> assurance that adequate clinical trials are in
> progress and will not be compromised, patients
> should have the right to obtain investigational
> drugs under expanded access INDs.*

*The existence of the committee as well as the approval of
AZT in record time are proof that the public can make a
difference.*

crazy! How can a handful of bureaucrats—unfeeling bureaucrats—tell us—the people who are paying the bills—that there
is nothing that can be done? In other countries, the search for
a treatment for AIDS is considered a *high* priority."

When these groups exerted pressure, when they got media
attention, when they exposed the weakness of the government's argument to the light of day—the rules were changed.

Now an AIDS patient who's dying can get anything he wants. However, a cancer patient who's dying can still be denied certain therapeutic agents because of the FDA's bureaucratic situation. The AIDS patients were vocal and found that there is strength in numbers. I'd like the cancer patients to become equally vocal. Considering the decades of research and the billions of taxpayer dollars that have been poured into cancer research, it's time for more people-oriented results.

My desire for people-oriented results led me to write this book to provide the information to the public. In the writing, I have perhaps jumped the gun a bit in relationship to procedure. I haven't yet had double-blind studies done on humans. I don't have five years' worth of anecdotal case histories. I am not involved in a project with a multimillion-dollar budget. What I have done, I believe, is find something that may be an important key in saving the lives of millions of people who would otherwise leave behind a grieving brother or sister, father or mother, husband or wife.

The information in this book is only a beginning. The studies are highly encouraging, but much more needs to be done. In fact, I believe that much more *must* be done. We need to know the whole truth, but without public pressure, that truth may be a very long time in coming.

With more women now in Congress and with breast cancer on the rise, I believe that it may very well be the women who will lead the movement to find the truth. Certainly, the early results of Dr. Roscoe L. Van Zandt's study (see page 99), in which eight of eight advanced breast cancer patients responded dramatically to shark-cartilage therapy, should be an eye opener. I believe it might cause women to reject orthodox medicine's pat comment that whole natural products are not worth in-depth studies.

You, too, can push for the truth. You, too, have it within yourself to help move the information in this book forward, to urge others to study shark cartilage further, to help ensure that shark-cartilage treatment is not "shelved" by a bureaucrat who is simply "following orders." Ultimately, the responsibility for your own health falls into your own hands. By joining our hands, we can make a difference.

A Further Word

As more and more people hear about shark cartilage's potential benefits as a cancer treatment and preventative, the commercial demand for shark cartilage is mushrooming. With increased media coverage, tens of thousands of people have rushed out to buy products being sold as shark cartilage. Although no product name was mentioned during the "60 Minutes" TV segment featuring shark cartilage, practically every product now on the market makes the claim, "as seen on '60 Minutes.'" The fact is, all the studies I initiated—studies that were discussed on "60 Minutes"—were conducted using one specific form of shark cartilage. My early work was done using a pure shark cartilage made in my kitchen in limited amounts. Since receiving my first patent, I have licensed only one company to manufacture the cartilage. This cartilage is produced under strict supervision to maintain the highest quality possible. I'm telling you this for one specific reason. If my work is to be judged on the basis of shark cartilage's performance, I most certainly do not want people using untested products that are masquerading as my shark cartilage.

It has taken me years to plan, test, and execute the development of a viable and safe product; I spent eight months perfecting the pulverization technique alone. There were years of leg work, animal studies, and clinical trials as documented in this book. It truly amazes me that so many companies seem to have accomplished in days what it took me years to do!

BUYERS BEWARE

The multitude of products flooding in from a number of countries—Japan, New Zealand, Scandinavia, and Australia—is burgeoning. Many of these products allude to the "60 Minutes" show, to this book, or to me. One company has produced a pamphlet entitled "Jaws of Life," which quotes freely from this book and from articles that I have authored. None of these products is, however, endorsed by me, by the producers of "60 Minutes," or by CBS. While these advertisements are misleading because of the implication of endorsement, it is more troubling that the products, offered under an array of labels, may be adulterated, ineffective, and perhaps even harmful.

One of the most telling examples of misguided manufacturing shortcuts can be seen in the processing of sharks. If you have seen the "60 Minutes" segment, you may recall the scenes showing and discussing the intensive amount of labor involved in removing and cleaning the shark cartilage. The cartilage must be cleaned of all flesh, and must be white in color so that the odor, flavor, and impurities are minimal and the biological activity high and undiluted. In order to achieve cartilage procurement and cleaning without raising costs to a prohibitive level, sharks must be fished in a nation where they are plentiful and where labor rates are modest. How can manufacturers in New Zealand and Australia—countries with the highest labor costs in the world—produce such a product? How can manufacturers in Japan and Scandinavia produce such a product with high labor costs and cold waters that limit the availability of local sharks? These discrepancies indicate that something is amiss about product claims of purity, high quality, and low price.

Furthermore, shark cartilage must be pulverized with extreme care so as not to render inactive the protein strands imbedded in a matrix of calcium and phosphorus salts and mucopolysaccharides. Pulverizing the inactive matrix is relatively easy; pulverizing the active protein strands simultaneously and effectively is most difficult. Most of the copycat products are long on matrix and almost devoid of active protein particles. Even if protein particles occur in the product, they may have been denatured (rendered inactive) by heat generated in an inadequate pulverization process.

One product on the market advertises itself as an "improved shark cartilage." This so-called "shark cartilage extract" is made in Japan, and its manufacturer has acknowledged in writing that the product is 45 percent dextrin; in other words, almost half the product is an inexpensive sugar derivative. I know of no evidence that would substantiate claims that dextrin or this diluted product are "improved," or even effective. Although removing some of the mineral salts (e.g., calcium and phosphorus) from whole shark cartilage would be beneficial, replacing them with sugar is laughable if not unscrupulous.

One Mexican clinic offers a product in powder or suppository form. "Alternatives," a well-known health newsletter, has suggested that there is a correlation between this product and serious intestinal upset. Another product, marketed by a multilevel marketing organization and an 800-number operation, claims to be shark cartilage, although it is yellowish instead of white in color. In addition, this product has a terrible odor and taste. Some of the products try to disguise their bad taste and rank odor, which may be caused by rotting or bacteria-laden remnants of shark flesh clinging to improperly cleaned cartilage, by adding flavoring.

KNOW WHAT YOU'RE DOING

Some uninformed people are recommending that cancer patients take three to six capsules of shark cartilage a day as a treatment. According to my work, this dose is meaningless. After the "60 Minutes" broadcast, hundreds of fifty- to one-hundred-capsule bottles of shark cartilage were sold. According to the research to date, a one-hundred-capsule bottle would comprise approximately a one-day dose. This is why patients in the current clinical trials are using shark cartilage in powder form. (For information on doses for various conditions, consult the index in the back of this book.) Although I have no data on preventative doses, I personally take ten 740-milligram capsules of shark cartilage daily. Hopefully, within the next year or so, research will begin on the protective uses of shark cartilage.

The discrepancies and confusion surrounding the marketing of shark cartilage led me to prepare this additional inset to "Sharks Don't Get Cancer." These problems have also convinced me of the need for a newsletter that would provide periodic updates of research on the most effective uses of shark cartilage. Those wishing to have their names added to the mailing list for this newsletter should call or write to:

Information Services
1–800–742–7534
P.O. Box 434
Short Hills, NJ 07078

Glossary

Acne. An inflammation of the oil glands that is characterized by pimples.

Adenocarcinoma. A malignant tumor of a gland.

Aflatoxins. A group of naturally occurring poisonous, carcinogenic factors produced by certain food molds.

AIDS. Acquired immune deficiency syndrome; a disease of the system that fights infection. It is thought to be caused by the HTLV-3 virus, which is spread through an exchange of body fluids.

Amino acid. An organic compound necessary for the formation of proteins and peptides, which are amino-acid chains. Some occur naturally in the body; some must be obtained from food.

Ampullae of Lorenzini. Skin pores in the shark's head region containing receptor cells sensitive to electric fields.

Analgesics. Pain-killing medications.

Angiogenesis. The development of new blood vessels.

Antiangiogenesis. The inhibition of the development of new blood vessels.

Antibody. A protein formed in the blood in reaction to certain substances that it then attacks and destroys.

Anticoagulant. A substance that retards or prevents the clotting of blood.

Antigen. A substance foreign to the body that stimulates the production of an antibody.

Apatite. A mineral made of calcium and phosphate. In sharks, it reinforces cartilage at stress points.

Arterioles. Small arteries.

Artery. One of the large blood vessels that carries oxygenated blood away from the heart.

Arthritis. An inflammation of the joints.

Articular cartilage. The cartilage in joints.

Assay. An analysis or examination.

Attenuated live-virus vaccine. Weakened living virus given orally or by injection to stimulate the development of immunity to infection by that virus.

Avascular. Without blood vessels.

AZT. The medication zidovudine, formerly called azidothymidine, which is most commonly used against AIDS.

Benign. Not malignant; harmless.

Biopsy. The removal from the body and microscopic examination of a small piece of living tissue.

Bony fishes. Fishes that have bones as opposed to just cartilage.

Bovine. Pertaining to an ox or cow.

Calcification. The impregnation of body tissues with calcium or calcium salts, which cause the tissues to harden.

CAM. Chicken chorioallantoic membrane.

CAM assay. A form of analysis in which chicken embryos are injected with a test substance and then analyzed to determine if the substance inhibits vascularization (see page 51).

Capillaries. The smallest blood vessels, at the far end of the circulatory system, linking arterioles and venules.

Capillary bed. A network of capillaries.

Capillary endothelium. The layer of cells lining the capillaries.

Carcinogen. A cancer-producing substance.

Carcinoma. A malignant tumor originally composed of epithelial cells.

Cartilage. A gristle-like supporting connective tissue.

Cell line. The "family line" of a tumor cell; the cells "parented" by a specific tumor cell.

Chorioallantoic membrane. A fetal membrane formed by the close association or fusion of two other embryonic membranes (the chorion and allantois).

Chondrocytes. Cartilage cells.

Clasper. The rodlike modification of the pelvic fins of male sharks. It is used during mating.

Collagen. The main supportive protein of bone, cartilage, and connective tissue.

Control group. The group of animals or people in a study that is left untreated and used as the standard against which the treated groups are judged.

Controlled trial. An organized, directed study or experiment in which control groups are used.

Cornea. The transparent structure covering the lens of the eye.

Corpus luteum. A yellow mass that appears in the place from which an egg has been discharged from the ovary.

Corticoid. A hormone produced in the adrenal cortex, which is the outer layer of the adrenal gland.

Denature. To change the characteristics of a protein by heating it or treating it with a chemical agent so that some of its original properties are diminished or eliminated.

Dermal denticles. Small sharp scales that cover the shark's skin.

Diabetic retinopathy. An eye disorder associated with diabetes in which the small blood vessels that transverse the retina dilate and rupture, leaving residues that usually impede vision.

DNA. Deoxyribonucleic acid; a large nucleic-acid molecule that is the carrier of genetic information, found mainly in the chromosomes.

Dorsal fin. The large triangular fin on the shark's back.

Double-blind study. A study in which neither the researchers nor the subjects know who is and is not receiving the substance being tested.

Duodenal ulcer. An ulcer in the duodenum, which is the first part of the small intestine.

Edema. Swelling of body tissues as the result of being filled with fluid.

Elasmobranchs. Sharks, rays, and skates; members of a subclass of the class Chondrichthyes.

Endothelial cells. The cells that make up the walls of blood vessels.

Endothelium. The layer of cells lining the heart and vessels of the circulatory system.

Enteritis. An inflammation in the lining of the bowels.

Enzyme. A chemical substance produced in the body that speeds up or causes a chemical reaction.

Epidemiologist. A person who studies the causes, development, and spread of epidemics.

Femoropatellar "degenerative" joint disease. A deterioration of the knee and thigh joints.

Fibrocartilage. The cartilage found between the back bones. It is the strongest type of cartilage and contains a great many white collagen fibers.

GAG. Glycosaminoglycan; a component of skin and of shark cartilage.

Gelatinize. To turn to gelatin or jelly.

Gills. The respiratory organ of fishes and other aquatic animals.

Glioblastoma multiforme. A fast-growing cancer of the brain or spinal cord that is made of glial (a type of nerve) cells.

Gold salts. A gold compound used for treating arthritis.

Heavy metals. Metals with a high molecular weight or high atomic number.

Heimlich maneuver. An emergency method for dislodging a piece of food or other object from the windpipe to prevent choking.

Hemangioma. A benign tumor that is composed of a continually growing blood pocket or mass of blood vessels.

Hemorrhagic necrosis. A process in which a tumor bleeds into itself, turns black, dries up, and dies.

Heparin. An acid mucopolysaccharide that prolongs the clotting time of whole blood. It occurs in a variety of tissues, most abundantly in the liver.

Histology. The study of minute anatomy; the observation through a microscope of normal and diseased cells and tissues.

Hodgkins. A malignant disease characterized by the progressive enlargement and inflammation of lymph tissues, particularly the spleen.

Hyaline cartilage. The gristly elastic cartilage that thinly covers the moving ends of bones, connects the ribs to the breastbone, and supports the nose, windpipe, and parts of the voice box. This type of cartilage is likely to harden in elderly people.

Hysterectomy. Surgical removal of all or part of the uterus.

Ichthyologist. A scientist who studies fishes.

Immunoglobulin. A protein, produced in animals, having antibody activity.

Immunosuppressant. A substance that suppresses the immune response to an antigen.

Infarct. An area of dead or damaged tissue resulting from the failure of blood to reach the affected part. Infarcts are commonly found in the heart muscle following heart attacks.

In vitro. In glass; refers to experiments performed in test tubes rather than on living organisms.

In vivo. Refers to experiments performed on living creatures.

Ischemic. Characterized by the loss of blood supply, usually due to some damage to the blood vessels.

Kaposi's sarcoma. A form of cancer in which irregular-shaped tumor cells cling to the linings of small blood vessels.

Killed-virus vaccine. Dead virus given orally or by injection to stimulate the development of immunity to infection by that virus.

Laser. "Light amplification by stimulated emission of radiation"; a distinct pencil-thin beam of pure, powerful light used for transmitting signals and for cutting everything from body tissues to thick metals.

Lateral-line system. A series of sensory canals along the sides of the shark's head and body. Hairlike receptors in the canals detect vibrations, pressure changes and waves, and movements in the water. Used for maintaining balance and detecting sound.

Lesion. A wound, injury, or other alteration in body tissue.

Leukemia. A cancer of the blood-forming tissues involving uncontrolled development of white blood cells.

Live-virus vaccine. *See* Attenuated live-virus vaccine.

Loading phase. The stage of treatment in which the patient or subject is given gradually larger doses of the medication or test substance to allow the body to adjust and to determine if there are any allergies.

Lymphoma. Any abnormal growth of lymphoid tissue.

Macula lutea. An area of the retina near the optic nerve that has special cones on which images must be focused for accurate sight to occur.

Macular degeneration. A condition in which leaking blood vessels under the central portion of the retina (the macula) cause damage and scarring that eventually lead to blindness.

Maintenance phase. The stage of treatment in which a desired effect has been achieved, and the patient or subject is given steady doses of the medication or test substance in order to maintain the effect.

Malignant. Refers to runaway growth that crowds out normal tissues.

Mandibular alveolitis. An extremely painful gum condition that sometimes follows tooth extractions; also known as "dry socket."

Melanoma. A dark-colored tumor of the skin that is usually malignant.

Metastasize. To spread to other places within the body.

Microscopy. Utilizing a microscope.

Microvessel. A very small blood vessel, specifically a capillary or venule.

Mucopolysaccharide. Any of a group of carbohydrates containing an amino sugar and uronic acid (a sugar acid). Mucopolysaccharides have been found to have an anti-inflammatory effect.

Necrosis. A condition characterized by the death of body tissues or cells that are still in place and surrounded by living tissue.

Neoplasm. A new growth in body tissues; a tumor. It can be malignant or benign.

Neovascular glaucoma. Glaucoma caused by neovascularization at the edge of the chamber containing the aqueous humor. Glaucoma is an increased pressure in the eyeball that produces defects in the field of vision.

Neovascularization. The formation of new blood vessels; a synonym for "angiogenesis."

Nictitating membrane. A membrane below the eyelid in many vertebrates that is capable of extending over the eyeball.

Nonsteroidal anti-inflammatory drugs (NSAIDs). Inflammation-fighting medications that do not contain steroids.

Osteoarthritis. A degenerative disease of the articular cartilage.

Palpate. To examine by touching.

Parenteral. "Outside the gut," as when medications are administered by routes other than the mouth, for instance, intravenously.

Pectoral fins. The large fins on the sides of the shark's body near the head.

Peptic ulcer. A lesion in the mucous membrane of the stomach or other part of the digestive system; also known as gastric ulcer.

Peritoneal. Relating to the peritoneum, the interior of the abdomen, more specifically the strong membrane that lines the abdomen and helps hold the internal organs in place.

Petri dish. A shallow glass or plastic dish with a loosely fitting, overlapping cover used for bacterial plate cultures and plant and animal tissue cultures.

Preload experiment. A type of experiment in which the test substance is administered prior to the introduction of the adverse condition.

Prevascular. Referring to the condition of an area before the development of blood vessels.

Primary cancer. The original cancer in a body in regards to site and type.

Prophylactic. Tending to prevent a disease.

Proteolytic enzymes. Enzymes that aid the breakdown of protein.

Pruritus ani. An intense chronic itching in the anal area caused by conditions such as a skin rash, hemorrhoids, pinworms, or psoriasis.

Psoriasis. A skin disorder characterized by reddish brown patches that become covered with silvery white or grayish scales of dead skin that eventually drop off.

Pulmonary embolism. A condition in which a lung artery is blocked by foreign matter such as air, fat, tumor tissue, or a blood clot.

Pulverize. To grind to a powder.

Retention enema. A procedure in which fluid is introduced into the rectum, held for as long as possible, and then expelled.

Retina. A membrane lining the inside of the eyeball and connected to the brain through the optic nerve.

Rheumatoid arthritis. An inflammatory disease primarily affecting the joints of the body.

Rheumatology. The study of diseases that cause inflammation in the joints, muscles, or fibrous tissue.

Salicylates. Medications made from salicylic acid. Aspirin is a salicylate.

Sarcoma. A malignant tumor on connective tissue.

Secondary tumor. Not the original tumor in a body.

Skeletal radiograph. An image, usually made by x-ray, showing where a radioactive substance is located.

Skin patch. An adhesive patch containing medication that is placed on the skin to allow the medication to be absorbed directly into the skin.

Sonography. A diagnostic tool in which an image is made of the body using transmitted and reflected acoustic (sound) waves.

Squamous cell cancer. A carcinoma composed principally of immature or undifferentiated cells on free surfaces or lining the vessels of the circulatory system.

Suppository. A medication formed into a solid cone or cylinder that is placed into the rectum, vagina, or urethra, where it melts and releases the medication directly into the system.

Synergistic. A combined effect that exceeds the sum of its parts.

Tail fin. The tail of the shark.

Tapetum lucidum. A structure located behind the retina of the shark's eye consisting of reflecting plates and used to enhance vision.

Teratogenicity study. A study to determine if a test substance administered to subjects produces physical defects in offspring conceived after the substance was administered.

Thrombosis. A condition in which a blood clot develops within a blood vessel.

Topical. Referring to a specific surface area of the body.

Toxicity study. A study to determine if a substance is toxic.

Tumor. A neoplasm; new tissue made of cells that grow in an uncontrolled manner.

Tumor marker. A substance in the body that has been connected to cancer but does not definitely indicate cancer.

Tumor necrosis factor. A substance or condition within cells that could cause a tumor to die.

Ulcer. A lesion on the skin or in a mucous membrane of the body.

Vaginectomy. Surgical removal of all or part of the vagina.

Vasculature. System of blood vessels; blood network.

Venous occlusion. A blockage in a vein.

Ventilatory capacity. Lung capacity.

Venule. A small vein that collects blood from a capillary.

Vertebrae. The bones or cartilaginous segments that compose the spinal column.

Vertebrate. An animal with a backbone.

Water suspension. A method of administering medication in which the dry medication is mixed (suspended) in water.

Xenograft. A procedure in which tissue is transplanted from one animal to an animal of a different species.

Yellow cartilage. The most elastic cartilage. It is found in the external ear, Eustachian tube, and throat as well as in other sites.

Bibliography

Angiogenesis

Azizkhan, Richard G., M.D.; Jane Clifford Azizkhan, Ph.D.; Michael Klagsbrun, Ph.D.; R. Clement Darling III, B.S.; Evan Rochman, B.S.; and Judah Folkman, M.D., F.A.C.S. "An Avascular Subpopulation of Chondrosarcoma Exhibits Limited Growth in Vivo and Is Unable to Stimulate Capillary Endothelial Cells in Vitro." *Surgical Forum* 32:424–426, 1981.

Blumberg, Neil. "Tumor Angiogenesis Factor: Speculations on an Approach to Cancer Chemotherapy." *Yale Journal of Biology and Medicine* 47:71–81, 1974.

Blumenson, Leslie E., and Irwin D.J. Bross. "A Possible Mechanism for Enhancement of Increased Production of Tumor Angiogenic Factor." *Growth* 40:205–209, 1976.

Brem, Henry, and Judah Folkman. "Inhibition of Tumor Angiogenesis Mediated by Cartilage." *Journal of Experimental Medicine* 141:427–439, 1975.

Brown, Robert A.; Jacqueline B. Weiss; Ian W. Tomlinson; Paul Phillips; and Shant Kumar. "Angiogenic Factor From Synovial Fluid Resembling That From Tumours." *The Lancet*, 29 March 1980, pp. 682–685.

Chaudhury, Triptesh; Michael P. Lerner; and Robert E. Nordquist. "Angiogenesis by Human Melanoma and Breast Cancer Cells." *Cancer Letters* 11:43–49, 1980.

Cohen, Samuel; Masae Tatematsu; Yoshitaka Shinohara; Keisuke Nakanishi; and Nobuyuki Ito. "Neovascularization in Rats During Urinary Bladder Carcinogenesis Induced by N-[4-(5-Nitro-2-furyl)-2-thiazolyl]formamide." *Journal of the National Cancer Institute* 65:145–147, 1980.

Crim, Joe William, and Robert A. Huseby. "Initial Events in the Vascularization of Day-Old Mouse Testes Implanted Into the Inguinal Mammary Gland Fat Pad: A Light Microscopic and Autoradiographic Study." *Microvascular Research* 12:141–156, 1976.

Crum, Rosa; Sandor Szabo; and Judah Folkman. "A New Class of Steroids Inhibits Angiogenesis in the Presence of Heparin or a Heparin Fragment." *Science* 230:1375–1378, 1985.

D'Amore, Patricia A., Ph.D. "Antiangiogenesis as a Strategy for Antimetastasis." *Seminars in Thrombosis and Hemostasis* 14:73–77, 1988.

D'Amore, Patricia, and Michael Klagsbrun. "Angiogenesis: Factors and Mechanisms" in *The Pathobiology of Neoplasia,* Alphonse E. Sirica, ed. New York: Plenum Publishing Corporation, 1989.

D'Amore, Patricia; Alicia Orlidge; and Ira M. Herman. "Growth Control in the Retinal Microvasculature" in *Progress in Retinal Research,* N. Osborne and J. Chader, eds. New York: Pergamon Press, 1988.

Eisenstein, Reuben, M.D.; Klaus E. Kuettner, Ph.D.; Carole Neapolitan, B.S.; Lawrence W. Soble, M.S.; and Nino Sorgente, Ph.D. "The Resistance of Certain Tissues to Invasion." *American Journal of Pathology* 81:337–346, 1975.

Ferguson, J.W., and A.C. Smillie. "Vascularization of Premalignant Lesions in Carcinogen-Treated Hamster Cheek Pouch." *Journal of the National Cancer Institute* 63, 1383–1391, 1979.

Folkman, Judah. "Antiangiogenesis" in *Biologic Therapy of Cancer,* Vincent T. DeVita, Jr., M.D.; Samuel Hellman, M.D.; and Steven A. Rosenberg, M.D., Ph.D., eds. Philadelphia: J.B. Lippincott Company, 1991.

———. "Tumor Angiogenesis: A Possible Control Point in Tumor Growth." *Annals of Internal Medicine* 82:96–100, 1975.

————. "Tumor Angiogenesis: Therapeutic Implications." *The New England Journal of Medicine* 285:1182–1186, 1971.

————. "The Vascularization of Tumors." *Scientific American* 234:59–73, 1976.

Folkman, Judah, and Michael Klagsbrun. "Angiogenic Factors." *Science* 235:442–447, 1987.

Folkman, Judah; Robert Langer; Robert J. Linhardt; Christian Haudenschild; and Stephanie Taylor. "Angiogenesis Inhibition and Tumor Regression Caused by Heparin or a Heparin Fragment in the Presence of Cortisone." *Science* 221:719–725, 1983.

Folkman, Judah; Paul B. Weisz; Madeleine M. Joullie; William W. Li; and William R. Ewing. "Control of Angiogenesis With Synthetic Heparin Substitutes." *Science* 243:1490–1493, 1989.

Gimbrone, Michael A., Jr.; Ramzi S. Cotran; Stephen B. Leapman; and Judah Folkman. "Tumor Growth and Neovascularization: An Experimental Model Using the Rabbit Cornea." *Journal of the National Cancer Institute* 52:413–427, 1974.

Goldsmith, Harry S., M.D.; Ann L. Griffith, Ph.D.; and Nicholas Catsimpoolas, Ph.D. "Lipid Angiogenic Factor From Omentum." *Journal of the American Medical Association* 252:2034–2036, 1984.

Huseby, Robert A.; Clyde Currie; Vincent A. Lagerborg; and Solomon Garb. "Angiogenesis About and Within Grafts of Normal Testicular Tissue: A Comparison With Transplanted Neoplastic Tissue." *Microvascular Research* 10:396–413, 1975.

Jacobs, Maryce M.; Phillippe Shubik; and Robert Feldman. "Influence of Selenium on Vascularization in the Hamster Cheek Pouch." *Cancer Letters* 9:353–357, 1980.

Knighton, David R.; Thomas K. Hunt; Heinz Scheuenstuhl; Betty J. Halliday; Zena Werb; and Michael J. Banda. "Oxygen Tension Regulates the Expression of Angiogenesis Factor by Macrophages." *Science* 221:1283–1285, 1983.

Kull, Frederick C., Jr.; David A. Brent; Indu Parikh; and Pedro Cuatrecasas. "Chemical Identification of a Tumor-Derived Angiogenic Factor." *Science* 236:843–846, 1987.

Kyozo, Tsukamoto, and Yukio Sugino. "Tumor Angiogenesis Activity in Clonal Cells Transformed by Bovine Adenovirus Type 3." *Cancer Research* 39:1305–1309, 1979.

Langer, Robert; H. Conn; J. Vacanti; C. Handenschid; and Judah

Folkman. "Control of Tumor Growth in Animals by Infusion of an Angiogenesis Inhibitor." *Proceedings of the National Academy of Sciences* 77:4331–4335, 1980.

Lee, Anne, and Robert Langer. "Shark Cartilage Contains Inhibitors of Tumor Angiogenesis." *Science* 221:1185–1187, 1983.

Lee, Kan-ei; Erdal Ertuk; Robert Mayer; and Abraham T.K. Cockett. "Efficacy of Antitumor Chemotherapy in C3H Mice Enhanced by the Antiangiogenesis Steroid, Cortisone Acetate." *Cancer Research* 47:5021–5024, 1987.

Mahadevan, Viswanath; Ian R. Hart; and Graham P. Lewis. "Factors Influencing Blood Supply in Wound Granuloma Quantitated by a New in Vivo Technique." *Cancer Research* 49:415–419, 1989.

Maione, Theodore E.; Gary S. Gray; Joan Petro; Anthony J. Hunt; Amy L. Donner; Susan I. Bauer; Helen F. Carson; and Richard J. Sharpe. "Inhibition of Angiogenesis by Recombinant Human Platelet Factor-4 and Related Peptides." *Science* 247:77–79, 1990.

Maiorana, Antonio, and Pietro M. Gullion. "Acquisition of Angiogenic Capacity and Neoplastic Transformation in the Rat Mammary Gland." *Cancer Research* 38:4409–4414, 1978.

Marx, Jean L. "Angiogenesis Research Comes of Age." *Science* 236:23–24, 1987.

Maugh, Thomas H., II. "Angiogenesis Inhibitors Link Many Diseases." *Science* 212:1374–1375, 1981.

McAuslan, B.R., and W. Reilly. "Selenium-Induced Cell Migration and Proliferation: Relevance to Angiogenesis and Microangiopathy." *Microvascular Research* 32:112–120, 1986.

Moses, Marsha A.; Judith Sudhalter; and Robert Langer. "Identification of an Inhibitor of Neovascularization From Cartilage." *Science* 248:1408–1410, 1990.

"Neovascularisation and Its Role in the Osteoarthritic Process." *Annals of the Rheumatic Diseases* 47:881–885, 1988.

Oikawa, H.; H. Ashino-Fuse; M. Shimamura; U. Koide; and T. Iwaguchi. "A Novel Angiogenic Inhibitor Derived From Japanese Shark Cartilage (I). Extraction and Estimation of Inhibitory Activities Toward Tumor and Embryonic Angiogenesis." *Cancer Letters* 51:181–186, 1990.

Phillips, Paul, and Shant Kumar. "Tumour Angiogenesis Factor (TAF) and Its Neutralisation by a Xenogeneic Antiserum." *International Journal of Cancer* 23:82–88, 1979.

Phillips, Paul; James K. Steward; and Shant Kumar. "Tumour Angiogenesis Factor (TAF) in Human and Animal Tumours." *International Journal of Cancer* 17:549–558, 1976.

"Protein Discovery: Blood Vessel Inducer Isolated, Cloned." *Chemical and Engineering News*, 30 September 1985, pp. 6–7.

Robertson, Nancy E.; Carolyn M. Discafani; Elizabeth C. Downs; Judith A. Hailey; Olga Sarre; Robert I. Runkle, Jr.; Thomas L. Popper; and Marian L. Plunkett. "A Quantitative in Vivo Mouse Model Used to Assay Inhibitors of Tumor-Induced Angiogenesis." *Cancer Research* 51:1339–1344, 1991.

Schreiber, Alain B.; Marjorie E. Winkler; and Rik Derynck. "Transforming Growth Factor-α: A More Potent Angiogenic Mediator Than Epidermal Growth Factor." *Science* 232:1250–1253, 1986.

Sidky, Younan A., and Ernest C. Borden. "Inhibition of Angiogenesis by Interferons: Effects on Tumor- and Lymphocyte-Induced Vascular Responses." *Cancer Research* 47:5155–5161, 1987.

Tamargo, Rafael J.; Robert A. Bok; and Henry Brem. "Angiogenesis Inhibition by Minocycline." *Cancer Research* 51:672–675, 1991.

Tatematsu, Masae; Samuel M. Cohen; Shoji Fukushima; Tomoyuki Shirai; Yoshitaka Shinohara; and Nobuyuki Ito. "Neovascularization in Benign and Malignant Urinary Bladder Epithelial Proliferative Lesions of the Rat Observed in Situ by Scanning Electron Microscopy and Autoradiography." *Cancer Research* 38:1792–1800, 1978.

Thompson, John A.; Kathryn D. Anderson; Judith M. DiPietro; James A. Zwiebel; Massimo Zametta; W. French Anderson; and Thomas Maciag. "Site-Directed Neovessel Formation in Vivo." *Science* 241:1349–1352, 1988.

Trapper, David, M.D.; Robert Langer, Sc.D.; A. Robert Bellows, M.D.; and Judah Folkman, M.D. "Angiogenesis Capacity as a Diagnostic Marker for Human Eye Tumors." *Surgery* 86:36–40, 1979.

Warner, T.F.C.S., and R.G. Krueger. "Perineural Angiogenesis in Mice Bearing Subcutaneous Tumors." *British Journal of Experimental Pathology* 59:282–287, 1978.

Wolff, J.R.; Ch. Goerz; Th. Bar; and F.H. Guldner. "Common

Morphogenetic Aspects of Various Organotypic Microvascular Patterns." *Microvascular Research* 10:373–395, 1975.

Arthritis

Griffin, Marie R., M.D., M.P.H.; Wayne A. Ray, Ph.D.; and William Schaffner, M.D. "Nonsteroidal Anti-Inflammatory Drug Use and Death From Peptic Ulcer in Elderly Persons." *Annals of Internal Medicine*, September 1988.

"Neovascularisation and Its Role in the Osteoarthritic Process." *Annals of the Rheumatic Diseases* 47:881–885, 1988.

Prudden, John F., and Leslie L. Balassa. "The Biological Activity of Bovine Cartilage Preparations." *Seminars in Arthritis and Rheumatism* 3:287–321, 1974.

Rejholee, V. "Long-Term Studies of Antiosteoarthritic Drugs: An Assessment." *Seminars in Arthritis and Rheumatism* 17:35–63, 1987.

Roth, Sanford H., M.D. "Nonsteroidal Anti-Inflammatory Drugs: Gastropathy, Deaths, and Medical Practice." *Annals of Internal Medicine* 109:353–354, 1988.

Cancer

Abramson, Maxwell, M.D.; Cheng-Chun Huang, Ph.D.; Robinson Schilling, M.D.; and Ronald G. Salome, B.S. "Collagenase Activity of the Oral Cavity and Larynx." *Annals of Otolaryngology* 84:158–163, 1975.

Algire, G.H., and H.W. Chalkley. "Vascular Reactions of Normal and Malignant Tissues in Vivo." *Journal of the National Cancer Institute* 6:73–85, 1945.

Andrews, Edmund L. "Patents: Tumor Treatment Made From Sharks." *The New York Times*, 15 February 1992.

Blumberg, Neil. "Tumor Angiogenesis Factor: Speculations on an Approach to Cancer Chemotherapy." *Yale Journal of Biology and Medicine* 47:71–81, 1974.

Brem, Henry, and Judah Folkman. "Inhibition of Tumor Angiogenesis Mediated by Cartilage." *Journal of Experimental Medicine* 141:427–439, 1975.

"Can Shark Cartilage Arrest Cancerous Tumors?" *Industry Week*, 1 April 1991.

Chaudhury, Triptesh; Michael P. Lerner; and Robert E. Nordquist.

"Angiogenesis by Human Melanoma and Breast Cancer Cells." *Cancer Letters* 11:43–49, 1980.

Cohen, Samuel; Masae Tatematsu; Yoshitaka Shinohara; Keisuke Nakanishi; and Nobuyuki Ito. "Neovascularization in Rats During Urinary Bladder Carcinogenesis Induced by N-[4-(5-Nitro-2-furyl)-2-thiazolyl]formamide." *Journal of the National Cancer Institute* 65:145–147, 1980.

D'Amore, Patricia A., Ph.D. "Antiangiogenesis as a Strategy for Antimetastasis." *Seminars in Thrombosis and Hemostasis* 14:73–77, 1988.

Dresden, Marc H.; Stephen A. Heilman; and Jimmy D. Schmidt. "Collagenolytic Enzymes in Human Neoplasms." *Cancer Research* 32:993–996, 1972.

Durie, Brian G.M.; Barbara Soehnlen; and John F. Prudden. "Antitumor Activity of Bovine Cartilage Extract (Catrix-S) in the Human Tumor Stem Cell Assay." *Journal of Biological Response Modifiers* 4:590–595, 1985.

Ferguson, J.W., and A.C. Smillie. "Vascularization of Premalignant Lesions in Carcinogen-Treated Hamster Cheek Pouch." *Journal of the National Cancer Institute* 63:1383–1391, 1979.

Fink, John M. *Third Opinion: An International Directory to Alternative Therapy Centers for the Treatment and Prevention of Cancer and Other Degenerative Diseases.* 2nd ed. Garden City Park, NY: Avery Publishing Group, 1992.

"Fishing for a Cancer Cure." *Discover*, September 1988.

Folkman, Judah. "How Is Blood Vessel Growth Regulated in Normal and Neoplastic Tissue?—G.H.A. Clowes Memorial Lecture." *Cancer Research* 46:467–473, 1986.

———. "Tumor Angiogenesis: A Possible Control Point in Tumor Growth." *Annals of Internal Medicine* 82:96–100, 1975.

———. "Tumor Angiogenesis: Therapeutic Implications." *The New England Journal of Medicine* 285:1182–1186, 1971.

———. "The Vascularization of Tumors." *Scientific American* 234:5973, 1976.

Folkman, Judah; Robert Langer; Robert J. Linhardt; Christian Haudenschild; and Stephanie Taylor. "Angiogenesis Inhibition and Tumor Regression Caused by Heparin or a Heparin Fragment in the Presence of Cortisone." *Science* 221:719–725, 1983.

Gimbrone, Michael A., Jr.; Ramzi S. Cotran; Stephen B. Leapman; and Judah Folkman. "Tumor Growth and Neovascularization: An Experimental Model Using the Rabbit Cornea." *Journal of the National Cancer Institute* 52:413–427, 1974.

Heuson, Jean-Claude; Jean-Lambert Pasteels; Nicole Legros; Jeanine Heuson-Stiennon; and Guy Leclercq. "Estradiol-Dependent Collagenolytic Enzyme Activity in Long-Term Organ Culture of Human Breast Cancer." *Cancer Research* 35:2039–2048, 1975.

Huseby, Robert A.; Clyde Currie; Vincent A. Lagerborg; and Solomon Garb. "Angiogenesis About and Within Grafts of Normal Testicular Tissue: A Comparison With Transplanted Neoplastic Tissue." *Microvascular Research* 10:396–413, 1975.

Kolata, Gina. "Powerful Hormone to Be Tested in War to Prevent Breast Cancer." *The New York Times*, 18 September 1991.

Kumar, Pat; Annalaura Erroi; A. Sattar; and S. Kumar. "Weibel-Palade Bodies as a Marker for Neovascularization Induced by Tumor and Rheumatoid Angiogenesis Factors." *Cancer Research* 45:4339–4348, 1985.

Kyozo, Tsukamoto, and Yukio Sugino. "Tumor Angiogenesis Activity in Clonal Cells Transformed by Bovine Adenovirus Type 3." *Cancer Research* 39:1305–1309, 1979.

Lane, I.W., Ph.D., and E. Contreras, Jr., M.D. "High Rate of Bioactivity (Reduction in Gross Tumor Size) Observed in Advanced Cancer Patients Treated With Shark Cartilage Material." *Journal of Naturopathic Medicine* 3:86–88, 1992.

Langer, R.; H. Brem; K. Falterman; M. Klein; and J. Folkman. "Isolation of a Cartilage Factor That Inhibits Tumor Neovascularization." *Science* 193:70–72, 1976.

Langer, Robert; H. Conn; J. Vacanti; C. Handenschid; and Judah Folkman. "Control of Tumor Growth in Animals by Infusion of an Angiogenesis Inhibitor." *Proceedings of the National Academy of Sciences* 77:4331–4335, 1980.

Laszlo, John, M.D. *Understanding Cancer*. New York: Harper and Row, Publishers, 1987.

Nicosia, Roberto F.; Ruy Tchao; and Joseph Leighton. "Angiogenesis-Dependent Tumor Spread in Reinforced Fibrin Clot Culture." *Cancer Research* 43:2159–2166, 1983.

Palca, Joseph. "Kaposi's Sarcoma Gives on Key Fronts." *Science* 255:1352–1354, 1992.

Pauli, Bendicht U., D.V.M.; Vincent A. Memoli, M.D.; and Klaus E. Kuettner, Ph.D. "Regulation of Tumor Invasion by Cartilage-Derived Anti-Invasion Factor In Vitro." *Journal of the National Cancer Institute* 67:65–73, 1981.

Phillips, Paul, and Shant Kumar. "Tumour Angiogenesis Factor (TAF) and Its Neutralisation by a Xenogeneic Antiserum." *International Journal of Cancer* 23:82–88, 1979.

Phillips, Paul; James K. Steward; and Shant Kumar. "Tumour Angiogenesis Factor (TAF) in Human and Animal Tumours." *International Journal of Cancer* 17:549–558, 1976.

Poole, A.R., and D.C. Williams. "In Vivo Effect of an Invasive Malignant Rat Tumour on Cartilage." *Nature* 214:1342–1343, 1967.

Prudden, John F. "The Treatment of Human Cancer With Agents Prepared From Bovine Cartilage." *Journal of Biological Response Modifiers* 4:551–584, 1985.

Renneker, Mark, ed. *Understanding Cancer*. Palo Alto, CA: Bull Publishing Company, 1988.

Sadove, Alan Michael, M.D., M.S., and Klaus E. Kuettner, Ph.D. "Inhibition of Mammary Carcinoma Invasiveness With Cartilage-Derived Inhibitor." *Surgical Forum* 28:499–501, 1977.

Sidky, Younan A., and Ernest C. Borden. "Inhibition of Angiogenesis by Interferons: Effects on Tumor- and Lymphocyte-Induced Vascular Responses." *Cancer Research* 47:5155–5161, 1987.

Simone, Charles B., M.D. *Cancer and Nutrition: A Ten-Point Plan to Reduce Your Risk of Getting Cancer*. Garden City Park, NY: Avery Publishing Group, 1992.

"Stopping the Progression of Cancer." *Alternatives for the Health Conscious Individual* 4:25–28, 1991.

Tatematsu, Masae; Samuel M. Cohen; Shoji Fukushima; Tomoyuki Shirai; Yoshitaka Shinohara; and Nobuyuki Ito. "Neovascularization in Benign and Malignant Urinary Bladder Epithelial Proliferative Lesions of the Rat Observed in Situ by Scanning Electron Microscopy and Autoradiography." *Cancer Research* 38:1792–1800, 1978.

Trapper, David, M.D.; Robert Langer, Sc.D.; A. Robert Bellows, M.D.; and Judah Folkman, M.D. "Angiogenesis Capacity as a Diagnostic Marker for Human Eye Tumors." *Surgery* 86:36–40, 1979.

Walker, Morton, D.P.M. "Therapeutic Effects of Shark Cartilage." *Townsend Letter for Doctors*, June 1989.

———. "Why Shark Cartilage Should Succeed Against Cancer and Other Pathologies." *Townsend Letter for Doctors*, November 1991.

Warner, T.F.C.S., and R.G. Krueger. "Perineural Angiogenesis in Mice Bearing Subcutaneous Tumors." *British Journal of Experimental Pathology* 59:282–287, 1978.

Weidner, Noel, M.D.; Joseph P. Semple, M.D.; William R. Welch, M.D.; and Judah Folkman, M.D. "Tumor Angiogenesis and Metastasis—Correlation in Invasive Breast Carcinoma." *New England Journal of Medicine* 324:1–8, 1991.

Cartilage

Abramson, Maxwell, M.D.; Cheng-Chun Huang, Ph.D.; Robinson Schilling, M.D.; and Ronald G. Salome, B.S. "Collagenase Activity of the Oral Cavity and Larynx." *Annals of Otolaryngology* 84:158–163, 1975.

Brem, Henry, and Judah Folkman. "Inhibition of Tumor Angiogenesis Mediated by Cartilage." *Journal of Experimental Medicine* 141:427–439, 1975.

"Can Shark Cartilage Arrest Cancerous Tumors?" *Industry Week*, 1 April 1991.

Caplan, Arnold I. "Cartilage." *Scientific American* 251:84–94, 1984.

Cherry, Laurence. "Artificial Skin: From Concept to Creation." *Reader's Digest*, September 1983.

Dresden, Marc H.; Stephen A. Heilman; and Jimmy D. Schmidt. "Collagenolytic Enzymes in Human Neoplasms." *Cancer Research* 32:993–996, 1972.

Eisenstein, Reuben, M.D.; Klaus E. Kuettner, Ph.D.; Carole Neapolitan, B.S.; Lawrence W. Soble, M.S.; and Nino Sorgente, Ph.D. "The Resistance of Certain Tissues to Invasion." *American Journal of Pathology* 73:765–774, 1973.

Heuson, Jean-Claude; Jean-Lambert Pasteels; Nicole Legros; Jeanine Heuson-Stiennon; and Guy Leclercq. "Estradiol-Dependent Collagenolytic Enzyme Activity in Long-Term Organ Culture of Human Breast Cancer." *Cancer Research* 35:2039–2048, 1975.

Irving, J.T., and J.D. Heeley. "The Effect of Enzyme Treatment Upon the Resorption of Scapular Implants." *Calcareous Tissue Research* 5:64–69, 1970.

Kuettner, Klaus E.; Harold Guenther; and Robert D. Ray. "Lysozyme in Preosscous Cartilage." *Calcareous Tissue Research* 1:298–305, 1968.

Kuettner, Klaus E.; Judith Hiti; Reuben Eisenstein; and Elvin Harper. "Collagenase Inhibition by Cationic Proteins Derived From Cartilage and Aorta." *Biochemical and Biophysical Research Communications* 72:40–46, 1976.

Lane, I.W., Ph.D., and E. Contreras, Jr., M.D. "High Rate of Bioactivity (Reduction in Gross Tumor Size) Observed in Advanced Cancer Patients Treated With Shark Cartilage Material." *Journal of Naturopathic Medicine* 3:86–88, 1992.

Lane, I. William, B.S., M.S., Ph.D. "The Medical Potential of Shark Cartilage." *The Natural Health Magazine*, October 1991.

————. "Shark Cartilage: Its Potential Medical Applications." *Journal of Advancement in Medicine* 4:263–271, 1991.

Langer, R.; H. Brem; K. Falterman; M. Klein; and J. Folkman. "Isolation of a Cartilage Factor That Inhibits Tumor Neovascularization." *Science* 193:70–72, 1976.

Lee, Anne, and Robert Langer. "Shark Cartilage Contains Inhibitors of Tumor Angiogenesis." *Science* 221:1185–1187, 1983.

Lindenbaum, Arthur, and Klaus E. Kuettner. "Mucopolysaccharides and Mucoproteins of Calf Scapula." *Calcareous Tissue Research* 1:1531165, 1967.

Moses, Marsha A.; Judith Sudhalter; and Robert Langer. "Identification of an Inhibitor of Neovascularization From Cartilage." *Science* 248:1408–1410, 1990.

Oikawa, H.; H. Ashino-Fuse; M. Shimamura; U. Koide; and T. Iwaguchi. "A Novel Angiogenic Inhibitor Derived From Japanese Shark Cartilage (I). Extraction and Estimation of Inhibitory Activities Toward Tumor and Embryonic Angiogenesis." *Cancer Letters* 51:181–186, 1990.

Pauli, Bendicht U., D.V.M.; Vincent A. Memoli, M.D.; and Klaus E. Kuettner, Ph.D. "Regulation of Tumor Invasion by Cartilage-Derived Anti-Invasion Factor in Vitro." *Journal of the National Cancer Institute* 67:65–73, 1981.

Poole, A.R., and D.C. Williams. "In Vivo Effect of an Invasive Malignant Rat Tumour on Cartilage." *Nature* 214:1342–1343, 1967.

Prudden, John F. "The Treatment of Human Cancer With Agents Prepared From Bovine Cartilage." *Journal of Biological Response Modifiers* 4:551–584, 1985.

Rosen, J.; W.T. Sherman; J.F. Prudden; and G.J. Thorbecke. "Immunoregulatory Effects of Catrix." *Journal of Biological Response Modifiers* 7:498–512, 1988.

Sadove, Alan Michael, M.D., M.S., and Klaus E. Kuettner, Ph.D. "Inhibition of Mammary Carcinoma Invasiveness With Cartilage-Derived Inhibitor." *Surgical Forum* 28:499–501, 1977.

Sakamoto, Seizaburo; Masako Sakamoto; Paul Goldhaber; and Melvin Glimcher. "The Inhibition of Mouse Bone Collagenase by Lysozyme." *Calcareous Tissue Research* 14:291–299, 1974.

"Stopping the Progression of Cancer." *Alternatives for the Health Conscious Individual* 4:25–28, 1991.

Walker, Morton, D.P.M. "Therapeutic Effects of Shark Cartilage." *Townsend Letter for Doctors*, June 1989.

———. "Why Shark Cartilage Should Succeed Against Cancer and Other Pathologies." *Townsend Letter for Doctors*, November 1991.

Sharks

Brown, Theodore W. *Sharks: The Silent Savages*. Boston: Little Brown and Company, 1973.

Budker, P. *The Life of Sharks*. London: Weidenfeld and Nicolson, 1971.

Castro, José I. *The Sharks of North American Waters*. College Station: Texas A and M University Press, 1983.

Clark, E. "Sharks Magnificent and Misunderstood." *National Geographic* 160:13–83, 1981.

Cousteau, Jacques-Yves, and Phillippe Cousteau. *The Shark: Splendid Savage of the Sea*. Garden City, NY: Doubleday and Company, 1970.

Ellis, Richard, and John McCosker. "What Fate Awaits the Great White Shark?" *Audubon*, September-October 1991.

Lineaweaver, Thomas H., III, and Richard H. Backus. *The Natural History of Sharks*. Philadelphia and New York: J.P. Lippincott Company, 1970.

Springer, Victor, and Joy P. Gold. *Sharks in Question: The Smithsonian Answer Book*. Washington, DC: Smithsonian Institution, 1989.

Vietmeyer, Noel. "Greatest Fish on Earth." *Reader's Digest*, July 1988.

Miscellaneous

Brown, Ronald. *Lasers: Tools of Modern Technology*. Garden City, NY: Doubleday and Company, 1968.

DiMasi, Joseph, Ph.D.; Ronald Hansen, Ph.D.; Henry G. Grabowski, Ph.D.; and Lewis Lasagna, M.D. "Cost of Invention in the Pharmaceutical Industry." *Journal of Health Economics* 10:107–142, 1991.

"Enforcing the Food, Drug, and Cosmetic Act." FDA Consumer Memo, DHEW Publication No. (FDA) 74-1018, 1974.

"FDA Recall Policies." FDA Consumer Memo, DHEW Publication No. (FDA) 79-1064, 1979.

Fettner, Ann Giudici, and William A. Check, Ph.D. *The Truth About AIDS: Evolution of an Epidemic*. New York: Holt, Rinehart and Winston, 1984.

Garrett, Laurie. "The Battle Over FDA Drug Policy." *Newsday*, 14 February 1989, Discovery Section Part III, p. 1.

Hinds, Michael deCourcy. "Speeding F.D.A. Drug Review." *The New York Times*, 22 September 1982.

Lasagna, Louis, M.D.; Theodore Cooper, M.D., Ph.D.; Gertrude Elion, D.Sc.; Emil Frei III, M.D.; Samuel Hellman, M.D.; Peter Barton Hutt, L.L.M.; Charles Leighton, M.D.; Thomas C. Merigan, Jr., Ph.D.; Henry C. Pitot, M.D., Ph.D.; and Dr. Elliott H. Stonehill. "Final Report of the National Committee to Review Current Procedures for Approval of New Drugs for Cancer and AIDS." Unpublished report of the President's Cancer Panel, National Cancer Program, National Cancer Institute, 15 August 1990.

Laurence, Clifford L. *The Laser Book: A New Technology of Light*. New York: Prentice Hall Press, 1986.

Mayer, Ken, M.D., and Hank Pizer. *The AIDS Fact Book*. Toronto: Bantam Books, 1983.

Patrusky, Ben. *The Laser: Light That Never Was Before*. New York: Dodd, Mead and Company, 1966.

"Policy on Importing Unapproved AIDS Drugs for Personal Use." FDA Talk Paper T88-51, 1988, 27 July 1988.

U.S., Office of Technology Assessment. *Assessing the Efficacy and Safety of Medical Technologies*. PB 286/929 (1978).

United States Patent Number 5,075,112, 24 December 1991.

Weiss, Rick. "Biomedicine: Uprooting A Major Cause of Blindness." *Science News* 138:207, 1990.

Williams, Greer. *Virus Hunters*. New York: Alfred A. Knopf, 1960.

About the Authors

Dr. I. William Lane received both his B.A. and M.A. in the field of Nutrition Science from Cornell University. He received his Ph.D. in Agricultural Biochemistry and Nutrition from Rutgers University. As a researcher, he studied and worked under two Nobel prize winners, Dr. James B. Sumner (winner in 1946) and Dr. Selman A. Waksman (winner in 1952).

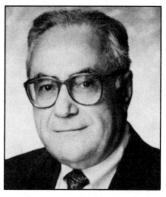

Entering industrial research, Dr. Lane first worked in poultry nutrition in association with Frank Perdue and Donald Tyson. From poultry-feed formulation, he moved into fishmeal production. Shifting into management, Dr. Lane joined W.R. Grace & Company as vice president, heading its Marine Resources Division, with operating plants in Peru, Chile, Brazil, Canada, and the United States.

After a successful decade in management, Dr. Lane was appointed by then-President Ronald Reagan to serve as a resource advisor to the newly emerging nation of Guinea. Upon his return from this mission, he became an independent consultant specializing in marine resources. Among his clients have been the United States Department of State, the Shah of Iran, the government of Morocco, and Taiyo, the largest fishing company in Japan. For the past ten years, Dr. Lane has pursued his interest in the benefits of shark cartilage as a healing agent.

Linda Comac received both her B.A. and M.A. in English from the City University of New York. She has taught English, journalism, and creative writing for more than two decades. As a freelance writer, her articles have appeared in numerous newspapers and journals. Having lost several friends to cancer, Ms. Comac has a very personal interest in the disease, an interest shared by her husband, a biochemist who has been conducting cancer research at various hospitals in New York City for almost twenty years.

Index

A

Acne, 127, 130
Ada, 121
Adam's apple, 11
Adenocarcinoma, 48
Aflatoxin B_1, 43
Aging, diseases associated with, 4, 111
AIDS (acquired immune deficiency syndrome)
    activists and impact on government, 145–149
    drugs for, 140, 147
    and Kaposi's sarcoma, 82, 83
    patients and drug research, 88
Allergic reaction, prevention of, 130
Alpizar
    Carlos Luís, 87–88, 119
    studies, 88, 119–120

Alternative therapies, orthodox medicine's view of, 139–145
American Cancer Society, 3
American Red Cross, 142
Analgesics as treatment for arthritis, 124
Angiogenesis
    and arthritis, 115, 117
    conditions based on, 4, 112–114
    inhibition in cartilage, reasons for, 42
    inhibition of, 40–41
    inhibition studies, 41–42, 44–45, 51, 66, 78–81
    inhibitor. *See* Angiogenesis inhibitor.
    and Kaposi's sarcoma, 83
    and metastasis, 49–50, 52–55, 57
    study, 49
    and tumor growth, 39, 40, 57

Other Books from Avery

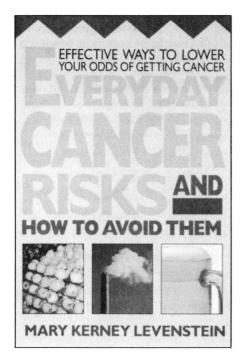

EVERYDAY CANCER RISKS & HOW TO AVOID THEM
Effective Ways to Lower Your Odds of Getting Cancer
Mary Kerney Levenstein

Contrary to what you may have heard, not everything gives you cancer. But because of all the conflicting information, many of us feel confused and overwhelmed. The fact is that there are many things you can do to reduce your risks. Everyday Cancer Risks and How to Avoid Them is a practical survival guide for everyone who's willing to take back control of his health.

Thoroughly researched, this comprehensive book details all the major cancer-causing problems you may unknowingly come face to face with in your home, food, work place, and lifestyle. The author then provides a list of specific options from which you can choose so that you can avoid, remove, or greatly lessen the risk of exposure. Names of key organizations, associations, and product suppliers are provided, should more information be necessary.

Don't let yourself become a statistic. Tip the odds back in your favor with Everyday Cancer Risks.

Trade Paperback, $11.95

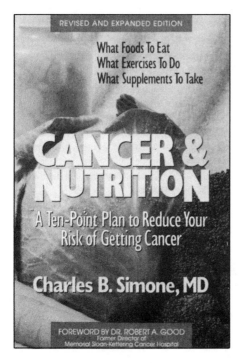

CANCER AND NUTRITION
A 10-Point Plan to Reduce Your Risk of Getting Cancer
Charles B. Simone

Based upon the latest scientifc research, Dr. Charles B. Simone tells you in straightforward language just what lifestyle adjustments and dietary changes you can make to significantly reduce the odds of getting cancer.

Cancer and Nutrition begins with a simple test that can tell you whether you or your loved ones are at great risk of getting cancer. The book goes on to explain what the highest risk factors are, and what the latest findings show to be anticancer agents. It tells you how to put together your own anticancer diet, what nutrients in foods can activate your body's natural defense system, what vitamins and minerals to take to best protect yourself, what exercises safeguard the body, and what sexual/social factors relate to cancer. It then provides you with ten easy-to-follow steps you can take to significantly reduce your chances of getting cancer.

Trade Paperback, $12.95

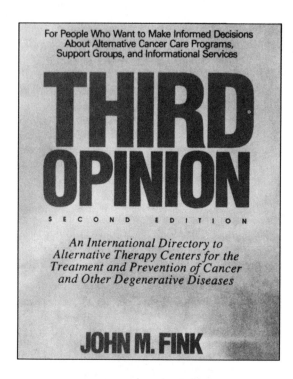

THIRD OPINION
An Int'l Directory to Alternative Therapy
Centers for the Treatment and Prevention of
Cancer and Other Degenerative Diseases
John M. Fink

Here, in an updated edition, is a comprehensive guide to the many alternative treatment
centers located throughout the world.
Everything you have to know—from addresses,
phone numbers, names, and prices, to philo-
sophical approaches and methods of treatment—is provided in a clear, easy-to-use for-
mat. Also included are the educational centers,
information services, and support groups that
may be of interest to the person looking for
alternative or adjunctive therapy.

Trade Paperback, $14.95

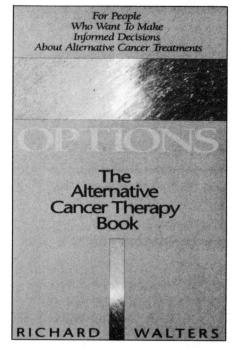

OPTIONS
The Alternative Cancer Therapy Book
Richard Walters

Alternative cancer therapies have helped thousands of "terminal" and "inoperable" cancer patients. Options covers a
wide spectrum of available alternative methods of treatment
from biologically-based approaches to immune-enhancing
treatments, dietary and nutritional regimens, herbal and
plant-based remedies, bioelectric medicine, and adjunctive
therapies, including information on recent experimental
advances in cancer treatment.

    This in-depth look at alternative therapies discusses how
each approach works, explains the scientific rationale
underlying each method, and presents clinical documenta-
tion of results. Options also includes guidelines for people
considering alternative treatments and gives detailed information on referral services that help patients choose the
combination of therapies best suited to their condition.

Trade Paperback, $13.95

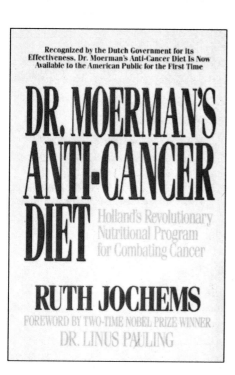

DR. MOERMAN'S ANTI-CANCER DIET
A Successful Nutrition Program
for Combating Cancer
Ruth Jochems with
Foreword by Dr. Linus Pauling

Cornelius Moerman first began work on his radical new diet for cancer in Holland in the 1930s. Now, sixty years later, the government of the Netherlands has approved his diet as a treatment against cancer. Ruth Jochems gives a clear account of how and why the diet works, detailing the combination of vitamins and minerals used, and the diet to follow.

His theory was based on one elementary idea—that the body's natural defenses are far more sophisticated than anything a laboratory could produce. Instead of concentrating treatment on just the tumor, he wanted to enhance the body's immune system so that the body could heal itself.

In his book, Jochems gives a clear account of how and why the diet works. He details the combination of vitamins and minerals to be used, and outlines the diet to follow. He also includes easy-to-follow recipes.

Trade Paperback, $9.95

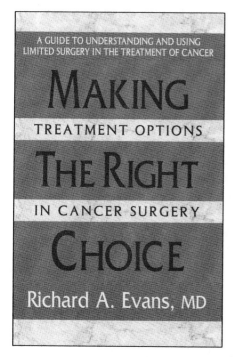

MAKING THE RIGHT CHOICE
Treatment Options in Cancer Surgery
Richard A. Evans, MD

To answer the many questions that cancer patients have when faced with surgery, Dr. Evans has written a complete and up-to-date guide to help them make the right choice—a choice based upon a clear understanding of the facts as they relate to today's research.

Dr. Evans is a board-approved surgeon who views conservative surgery—surgery that removes the least amount of tissue possible—as a viable option for numerous types of cancer. He begins his book by discussing how cancer surgery has evolved, how the training of surgeons has been carried out, and why the profession has been slow to change its procedures. He then looks at cancer—what it is, how it spreads, and how it can be contained. In Section Two, Dr. Evans takes a look at ten cancers that he thinks can be better treated with conservative surgery, from how each spreads to evaluations of treatments based upon the cancer's stages.

Trade Paperback, $14.95

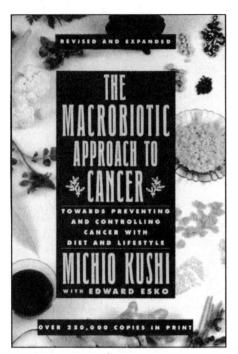

Trade Paperback, $9.95

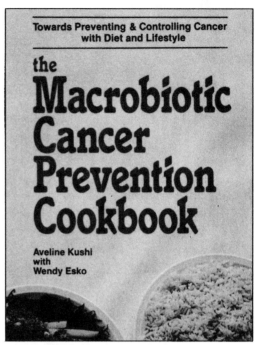

Trade Paperback, $9.95

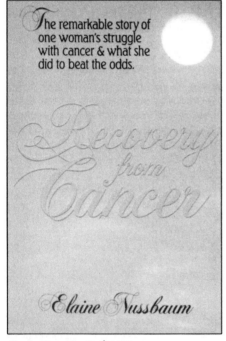

Trade Paperback, $9.95

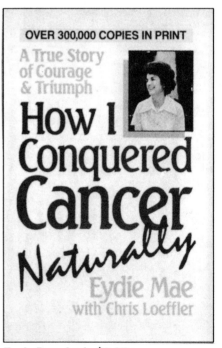

Trade Paperback, $9.95

Available at your local bookseller.
For a complete catalog of our books, call us at **1-800-548-5757**.